HIV/AIDS in Sub-Saharan Africa

Also by Adrian Flint

TRADE, POVERTY AND THE ENVIRONMENT: The EU, Cotonou and the African-Caribbean-Pacific Bloc

HIV/AIDS in Sub-Saharan Africa

Politics, Aid and Globalization

Adrian Flint

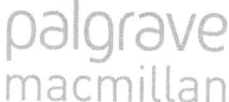

palgrave
macmillan

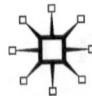
First published 2011 by
PALGRAVE MACMILLAN

Palgrave Macmillan in the UK is an imprint of Macmillan Publishers Limited, registered in England, company number 785998, of Houndmills, Basingstoke, Hampshire RG21 6XS.

Palgrave Macmillan in the US is a division of St Martin's Press LLC, 175 Fifth Avenue, New York, NY 10010.

Palgrave Macmillan is the global academic imprint of the above companies and has companies and representatives throughout the world.

Palgrave® and Macmillan® are registered trademarks in the United States, the United Kingdom, Europe and other countries

ISBN 978-0-230-22142-0   hardback

This book is printed on paper suitable for recycling and made from fully managed and sustained forest sources. Logging, pulping and manufacturing processes are expected to conform to the environmental regulations of the country of origin.

A catalogue record for this book is available from the British Library.

A catalogue record for this book is available from the Library of Congress.

10   9   8   7   6   5   4   3   2   1
20   19   18   17   16   15   14   13   12   11

Transferred to Digital Printing in 2014

In memory of Victor Flint,
Margaret Tunnell and William Tunnell

Contents

List of Tables and Maps

Tables

Maps

Acknowledgements

There are a number of people whom I would like to thank for helping to bring this book to fruition. First and foremost, for her tireless editing and advice, I would like to say thank you to Dr Jill Payne, whose efforts went well above and beyond the call of duty. I would also like to thank my colleagues at the Department of Politics, University of Bristol, for their encouragement and for giving me the benefit of their experience – in particular, I would like to thank Professor Sarah Childs for her comments on earlier drafts and Professors Mark Duffield and Terrell Carver for their patient advice. The Department of Politics has been generous in its support of my research, especially with regard to the funding of my field-work in South Africa in early 2009. For this, I am extremely grateful.

This book has been influenced heavily by my interaction with the Masters students who have taken my 'Politics of HIV/AIDS in Africa' unit over the past few years. Their debates, which frequently spilled out of the classroom and onto the pavement, forced me to continually rethink my position on a number of issues. I wish them, focused as they all are on making a difference in the 'real' world, all the best in their future careers.

The success of my South African fieldwork was due largely to the extraordinary hospitality and openness of the staff of various NGOs, faith organizations and youth groups. Numerous organizations, some of whom received little advance notice of my visits, gave freely of their time and experience, and for that I am greatly indebted to them. In particular, I would like to thank Zininzi Mpurwana and Pat Flint of REHAB (East London), Dr Ethne Schaefer and the staff of the Sophumelela Clinic (Inc), members of the Women in Partnership Against AIDS initiative, and Kazeka Somhlahlo of the Ikhwezi Lokusa Wellness Centre.

The Church of the Province of South Africa (Grahamstown Diocese) was exceptionally accommodating. The Very Rev Andrew Hunter, Dean of the Cathedral, facilitated a number of introductions to church groups involved in treating people living with HIV/AIDS (and gave me lunch). When I appeared at the Raphael Centre in Grahamstown, the staff, who had every right to instruct me to leave and book an appointment, instead could not have been more welcoming and obliging. Noelene Arende, the HIV/AIDS Co-ordinator for the Diocese, was a similarly patient font of knowledge. I would also like to thank Canon Louis Flint and the congregation of the Parish of St Luke the Evangelist outside East London for their time. I am especially grateful for the insights, frankness and good humour of the St Luke's youth groups. I am grateful, too, to Bishop Philip Le Feuvre for his responses to my questions.

Many people living with HIV/AIDS were prepared to talk to me about their experiences. In the interests of confidentiality, I am unable to name any of them here, but I would like them all to know how much I admire their steadfast refusal to be either cowed or defined by their HIV-positive status.

Finally, thank you to Helen McClure for the cover photograph.

List of Acronyms and Abbreviations

ABC	Abstain, Be Faithful, 'Condomize'
ACP	AIDS Control Programme
AIDS	Acquired Immunodeficiency Syndrome
ARV	Antiretroviral
CAFOD	Catholic Agency for Overseas Development
CATW	Coalition against Trafficking in Women
CCM	Country Coordinating Mechanisms
CDC	Centre for Disease Control
CEDAW	Convention on the Elimination of all forms of Discrimination against Women
CEFIKS	Centre for Indigenous Knowledge Systems
CGE	(South African) Commission on Gender Equality
CMMB	Catholic Medical Mission Board
CRS	Catholic Relief Services
DEVAW	Declaration on the Elimination of Violence against Women
DRB	(Ugandan) Domestic Relations Bill
DRC	Democratic Republic of Congo
FBO	Faith-based Organization
FDA	(US) Food and Drug Administration
GAO	Government Accountability Office
GATT	General Agreement on Tariffs and Trade
HIV	Human Immunodeficiency Virus
HRW	Human Rights Watch
ICTJ	International Center for Transitional Justice
IGLHRC	International Gay and Lesbian Human Rights Commission
IHV	Institute of Human Virology
IKS	Indigenous Knowledge System
IMA	Interchurch Medical Assistance
IPV	Intimate Partner Violence
LDC	Least Developed Countries
LFA	Local Fund Agent
MAP	(World Bank) Multi-Country HIV/AIDS Program for Africa
MCC	Medicines Control Council

MMM	Medical Missionaries of Mary
MSF	Médecins Sans Frontières
NGO	Non-Governmental Organization
NIAID	National Institute of Allergy and Infectious Diseases
NME	New Molecular Entity
OECD	Organization for Economic Cooperation and Development
PEP	Post-Exposure Prophylaxis
PEPFAR	(US) President's Emergency Plan for AIDS Relief
PhRMA	Pharmaceutical Research and Manufacturers of America
PMA	Pharmaceutical Manufacturers Association
PR	Principal Recipient
RAPCAN	Resources Aimed at the Prevention of Child Abuse and Neglect
SADC	Southern African Development Community
SAPS	South African Police Service
SIV	Simian Immunodeficiency Viruses
STI	sexually-transmitted infections
TAC	Treatment Action Campaign
TAWG	Tanga AIDS Working Group
THETA	Traditional and Modern Health Practitioners Together against AIDS
TRIPS	(WTO) Trade Related Aspects of Intellectual Property Rights
UN	United Nations
UNAIDS	United Nations Joint Programme on HIV/AIDS
UNCTAD	United Nations Conference on Trade and Development
UNDP	United Nations Development Programme
USTR	United States Trade Representative
WHO	World Health Organization
WTO	World Trade Organization
WWF	World Wildlife Fund

Introduction

In sub-Saharan Africa, HIV/AIDS has never been 'simply' about either health or development. More than anything, it has been about politics and governance at the national, regional and international level. With HIV/AIDS at the heart of the 'African Crisis' – in 2009, life expectancy in Lesotho, Mozambique and Zambia fell below the 45 year mark – governments, policymakers and NGOs, as well as students of African Politics and History, and Economics, Development, International Relations, Globalization and Gender Studies, face a series of dilemmas where response is concerned. *HIV/AIDS in Sub-Saharan Africa: Politics, Aid and Globalization* explains how issues of politics and governance lie at the heart of understanding and combating HIV/AIDS.

A book that is continental in scope was always going to be difficult to write. It is easy to succumb to over-reductionism and generalization and, frankly, to be left feeling that one has bitten off more than one can chew. The experience of HIV/AIDS is by no means consistent throughout Africa. North Africa has had little acquaintance with it. West and Central Africa have experienced limited effects. East Africa suffered heavily during the early stages of the pandemic but appears to have stabilized. Southern Africa currently bears the brunt of it (see Table 0.1).

As a lecturer on the politics and history of sub-Saharan Africa, I have struggled to find, let alone recommend, general historical and political texts that attempt a continental focus. There are exceptions: Bill Freund's (1998) excellent *The Making of Contemporary Africa: The Development of African Society Since 1800*, originally published in 1984, Martin Meredith's (2006) *The State of Africa: A History of Fifty Years of Independence*,[1] Alex Thomson's (2010) *An Introduction to African Politics*, Peter Schraeder's (2004) *African Politics and Society: A Mosaic in Transformation* and William

Table 0.1   HIV Prevalence Rates, Selected African Countries

Country	Prevalence (%) Adults 15–49	Country	Prevalence (%) Adults 15–49
Angola	2.1	Nigeria	3.1
Benin	1.3	Rwanda	2.8
Botswana	23.9	Senegal	1.0
Congo	3.5	Somalia	0.5
Eritrea	1.3	South Africa	18.1
Ethiopia	2.0	Swaziland	26.1
Gambia	0.9	Tanzania	6.2
Ghana	1.9	Togo	3.3
Guinea-Bissau	1.8	Uganda	5.4
Ivory Coast	3.9	Zambia	15.2
Mozambique	12.5	Zimbabwe	15.3
Namibia	15.3		

Source: (UNAIDS 2008d)

Tordoff's (2002) *Government and Politics in Africa*. In terms of colonial history, Thomas Pakenham's (1992) monolithic study, *The Scramble for Africa*, remains one of the few dedicated academic texts on the subject despite first being published in 1991. The fact that Muriel Chamberlain's (1999) *The Scramble for Africa*, originally published in 1974, is still in circulation as a recommended text demonstrates how little material of this nature is available.

A similar situation exists where HIV/AIDS is concerned. From the relative paucity of relevant titles within the academic literature, the difficulties inherent in adopting a continental, 'big picture' approach are apparent. The bulk of the academic material on HIV/AIDS tends to focus on either specific countries or regions, for example Pieter Fourie's (2006) *The Political Management of HIV and AIDS in South Africa: One Burden Too Many?* and Kerry Cullinan and Anso Thom's (2009) *The Virus, Vitamins and Vegetables: The South African HIV/AIDS Mystery*, or specific issues, including power (De Waal 2006), gender (Boesten and Poku 2009) and culture (Susser 2009). The fact that so many texts on HIV/AIDS in Africa tend to be edited works rather than monographs also speaks to the difficulties associated with generating a continental perspective. That being said, recent years have seen the publication of a number of highly notable monographs on HIV/AIDS: John Iliffe's (2006) *The African Aids Epidemic: A History*, Tony Barnett and Alan Whiteside's (2006) *AIDS in the Twenty-First Century: Disease and Globalization*, Amy Patterson's (2006) *The Politics of AIDS in Africa* and Alexander Rödlach's (2006) *Witches, Westerners and HIV: AIDS and Cultures of Blame in Africa*.

'Big picture' monographs are by no means necessarily superior to more focused studies. Nuance tends to be the first victim of any broad-based approach; the latter can paint a monolithic picture of a continent that does not, in effect, exist. However, reference to an 'African AIDS Crisis' is by no means unwarranted, and it may be that a general consideration of different states' differing experiences of the disease can speak to both theorists concerned with understanding the pandemic, and policymakers charged with containing and rolling it back.

In much the same way that famines are rarely 'acts of God', the spread of HIV/AIDS throughout Africa has not been wholly an act of nature. In fact, conspiracy theorists aside, there are those who would argue that the pandemic is iatrogenic in origin and therefore 'manmade', its emergence a result of mid-twentieth-century colonial-era vaccination policies. Be that as it may, the virulent escalation of the pandemic can be viewed as a clear-cut failure of governance across much of sub-Saharan Africa. In terms of combating HIV/AIDS, African political leadership has historically, with few exceptions, been poor and, in some cases, lamentable. In most instances, political elites chose simply to ignore the problem, which only served to exacerbate general uncertainty and stigmatize sufferers. Some elites' refusal to engage with and 'own' state responses to HIV/AIDS can be understood to be a consequence of the existence of strong donor programmes, particularly the United States' President's Emergency Plan for AIDS Relief (PEPFAR), the Global Fund to Fight AIDS, Tuberculosis and Malaria (Global Fund), and the World Bank's Multi-Country HIV/AIDS Program for Africa (MAP). However, these initiatives, all post-2000 in origin, postdate the onset of the HIV/AIDS crisis.

Two countries stand at opposite ends of the spectrum with respect to HIV/AIDS political leadership: Uganda and South Africa. While Uganda is generally viewed as a success story, South Africa's record has been met with concern and disbelief. The international donor response to the African situation has also been mixed. The generation of HIV/AIDS funding was slow for much of the 1980s and 1990s and it was close to two decades after the identification of HIV/AIDS before donors finally began to take seriously the funding of measures to combat what was by then a full-blown pandemic. The creation of PEPFAR, the Global Fund and MAP finally pushed HIV/AIDS to the forefront of the international development agenda.

Is Africa a special case?

The basic facts about HIV/AIDS in sub-Saharan Africa are these: according to 2008 data from the Joint United Nations Programme on HIV/AIDS

(UNAIDS 2009a), on a global level there are an estimated 33.4 million people living with HIV/AIDS, of whom 67 percent (over 22 million) are African. Over 70 percent of all deaths from AIDS occur in sub-Saharan Africa. Globally, of the estimated two million children under the age of 15 infected with HIV/AIDS, 90 percent (1.8 million) are from countries in sub-Saharan Africa (UNAIDS 2008a, 2008b). Moreover, estimates suggest that, as of 2008, at least 12 million African children have lost at least one parent to AIDS (UNAIDS 2008b). However, as demonstrated in Table 0.1, these figures belie considerable disparities across the continent; the burden of HIV/AIDS is by no means shared evenly (see Map 0.1).

The pattern and course of the HIV/AIDS in the sub-continent differ considerably from its incidence in other parts of the world. In sub-Saharan Africa, it is spread chiefly through heterosexual transmission or from mother to child, whereas in other regions it is generally confined to 'high risk' groups – in particular, men who have sex with men, intravenous drug users and sex workers (UNAIDS 2008b). Notable, too, is the fact that outwith Africa the distribution of HIV/ AIDS between men and women is broadly 50/50, whereas in sub-Saharan Africa it is women who are disproportionately affected. Nearly 60 percent of sub-Saharan African HIV/AIDS sufferers are female (UNAIDS 2008b).

One of the questions I address here is why certain parts of Africa, especially southern Africa, have been so unduly affected by HIV/AIDS. Should HIV/AIDS be viewed simply as part of the continental-wide 'African Crisis', characterized by high levels of poverty, poor leadership, political instability, civil strive, disease, famine and environmental degradation, or should it be pigeon-holed as a wholly separate phenomenon and addressed as such? While former South African President Thabo Mbeki has been confronted over many of his pronouncements on HIV/ AIDS, certain aspects of his argument ring very true indeed:

> The world's biggest killer and the greatest cause of ill-health and suffering across the globe is listed almost at the end of the International Classification of Diseases. It is given the code Z59.5 – extreme poverty. Poverty is the main reason why babies are not vaccinated, why clean water and sanitation are not provided, why curative drugs and other treatments are unavailable and why mothers die in childbirth. It is the underlying cause of reduced life expectancy, handicap, disability and starvation. Poverty is a major contributor to mental illness, stress, suicide, family disintegration and substance abuse. Every year in the developing world 12.2 million children under 5 years die, most of them from causes which could be prevented for just a few US cents per child. They die largely because of world indifference, but most of

Map 0.1   A Global View of HIV Infection

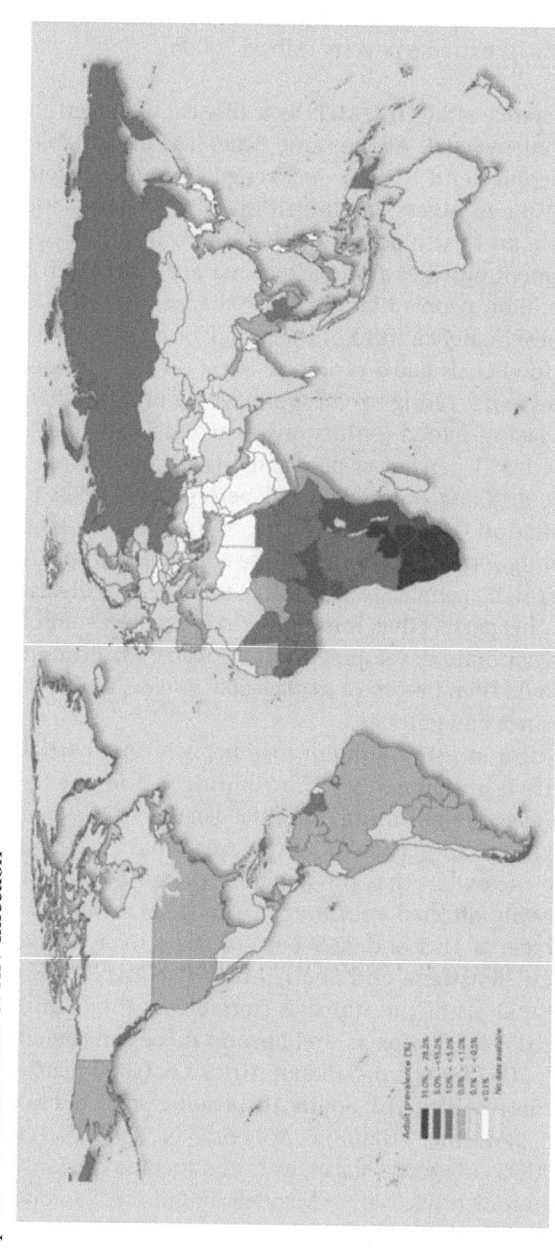

Source: (UNAIDS 2008d)

all they die because they are poor ... The world's biggest killer and the greatest cause of ill health and suffering across the globe, including South Africa, is extreme poverty (Mbeki 2000b).

Mbeki's insistence that HIV/AIDS is a disease of poverty was – and remains – controversial. At the same time, it is undeniable that malnourished people tend to have weakened immune systems and are more susceptible to illness: 'malnutrition in all its forms increases the risk of disease and early death' (WHO 2001). In a nutshell, Mbeki's poverty argument provides a simple explanation for HIV/AIDS in Africa; nearly 300 million people living in sub-Saharan Africa are 'chronically hungry', approximately a third of the population (UNCTAD 2009). The 2008 global food crisis had a profound effect on the continent, driving up food prices and creating severe shortages. As of 2010, there were still 36 countries facing 'a food security crisis', of which 21 were African (UN 2010). Similarly, 51 percent of people living in sub-Saharan Africa lack access to safe drinking water, while 41 percent lack access to adequate levels of sanitation (WWF 2002). A lack of the basic necessities – food, water and sanitation – across much of the continent means that, with or without HIV/AIDS, people are vulnerable to ill-health, disease and early death. From this perspective, it is logical to argue in favour of the prioritization of economic development and poverty eradication in Africa. HIV/AIDS would then become a manageable disease, in the way that it is in North America and Europe.

However, neat as this argument may be, it is only partially correct. While poverty is undoubtedly a contributing factor, it is by no means the sole or even determining variable. Firstly, other economically-deprived regions – in particular, South Asia – have not suffered from HIV/AIDS to the extent that sub-Saharan Africa has. Secondly, two of the most heavily affected countries in sub-Saharan Africa, with adult prevalence rates of 18.1 and 23.9 percent respectively, are also two of the wealthiest: Botswana and South Africa (UNAIDS 2008b). Furthermore, close analysis of the statistics from across the continent makes it clear that HIV/AIDS impacts well beyond those considered 'poor and uneducated'; 200,000 of sub-Saharan Africa's 650,000 teachers are predicted to die from AIDS, with South Africa alone predicted to lose nearly 45,000 such personnel (National Academy of Public Administration 2006). HIV/AIDS cuts across status, class and income barriers, with high-profile African leaders like Nelson Mandela and former Zambian President Kenneth Kaunda both having lost children to it. In addition, the fact that 58 percent of those infected are women (WHO 2003) cannot be accounted for simply in terms of poverty. Further factors must be considered.

What besides poverty, then, might make Africa 'different' where HIV/ AIDS is concerned? A number of issues are potentially pertinent in this respect. Firstly, the African origins of the disease and the fact that it went undetected for decades means that it had the opportunity to spread largely unnoticed through the countries of West and Central Africa. While determining a date for the origins of HIV/AIDS has proven difficult, the earliest confirmed case dates back to a serum sample collected by a malaria researcher in Leopoldville in the Congo in 1959 that suggests, at minimum, a mid-twentieth century origin (Iliffe 2006). A Los Alamos National Laboratory study produced a 'look-back' estimate for one of the key strains of HIV, HIV-1, to 1930. Allowing for a margin of error of 20 years on either side, this puts the origin of HIV at between 1910 and 1950 (Burr *et al* 2001). Its exact origins are arguably less important than combating its spread, but its genesis nonetheless provides a number of talking points. It is now generally accepted that HIV has its origins in a group of similar viruses affecting chimpanzees and other primates: Simian Immunodeficiency Viruses (SIV). Science is now largely of the view that the two key strains of HIV (HIV-1 and HIV-2) originated in chimpanzee and sooty mangabey, *Cercocebus (torquatus) atys*, populations in Western Equatorial Africa (Sharp *et al* 2000). Quite how SIV 'jumped' the species barrier during the early to mid-twentieth century is, however, hotly contested. Diseases regularly jump the species barrier and some of humanity's most common ailments, including measles, smallpox, tuberculosis, typhus, plague, Dengue fever, yellow fever and all types of influenza, had animal origins. There are a number of HIV-origin hypotheses; some arguments emphasize a 'natural' explanation, while others favour an iatrogenic origin.

The 'cut hunter' theory proffers the view that hunters butchering 'bush meat' became infected with SIV *via* contaminated blood, with the virus then mutating into HIV (Moore 2004). However, the fact that humans have been hunting chimpanzees and sooty mangabeys for millennia engenders questions as to why that jump did not occur earlier.

The hotly-disputed iatrogenic theories point to some form of human intervention, either in the origins of the disease, its dissemination, or both. In 1999, Edward Hooper (1999) proposed that SIV was introduced into the human population as a result of the mass polio vaccine programmes in effect in West and Central Africa during the colonial era. In *The River* he argued that the live vaccines were grown in chimpanzee tissue infected with SIV. While this theory was ostensibly disproven when a sample of the vaccine was discovered and found to be free of the virus, the mass vaccination programmes of this era may yet offer an explanation for the spread of HIV (Marx *et al* 2001). In the 1950s and

1960s, approximately 35 million people in Central Africa were vaccinated against yaws alone.[2] The high cost of syringes and poor facilities meant that much of this work was undertaken with contaminated needles. If HIV was present in small pockets of these regions, such blood transfers could quite conceivably have resulted in a rapid spread of the disease.

That HIV was not properly identified until 1982 meant that there was little that West and Central African states could have done to prevent the growing pandemic in those regions. This alone could arguably explain the disproportionate effect that the disease has had in sub-Saharan Africa. However, once HIV was identified, African governments were indisputably slow to react. Southern African governments were particularly slow. By the mid-1980s, HIV's inexorable progress south was clearly evident (see Map 0.2) – and so was the choice of many governing authorities to ignore the warning signs.

South Africa was notably culpable in this regard, despite warnings of an impending pandemic from medical practitioners and researchers from as early as 1988 (for example, see Ijsselmuiden *et al* 1988; Hunt 1989; Zwi and Bachmayer 1990). While extended indulgence in 'if only' scenarios is unhelpful, a degree of analysis is nonetheless important to a broader understanding of 'why Africa?' And, in particular, 'why southern Africa?'

Political leadership and HIV/AIDS

The record of African political elites in confronting and combating HIV has improved greatly of late, but there is no doubt that in the past it has been extremely poor. In sub-Saharan Africa, the majority of elites disregarded the disease for much of the 1980s and 1990s, despite evidence from agencies like the WHO that suggested that a potential pandemic was at hand. The Nigerian situation is just one example of an opportunity missed. The country's first National Conference on AIDS was only convened in December 1998, even though the first confirmed case of HIV in Nigeria dates back to 1985 (Oppong and Agyei-Mensah 2003). Similarly, it has been argued that, in the late 1980s, the Malawian government's National AIDS Committee was viewed by elites as a vehicle for obtaining access to increased levels of aid and foreign exchange (Lwanda 2003). The government of Cameroon has similarly been accused of being more interested in acquiring donor funding than actively engaging with the pandemic, while Côte d'Ivoire cut health spending from an already low figure of 1.5 percent of GDP in 1990 to just 1 percent in 2001 (Eboko 2005). The Zimbabwean government, too, for much of the 1990s largely ignored the burgeoning pandemic, effectively cutting its HIV/ AIDS expenditure towards the end of the decade (Batsell 2005).[3] However, there have been

Map 0.2 Adult Prevalence (1990–2007)

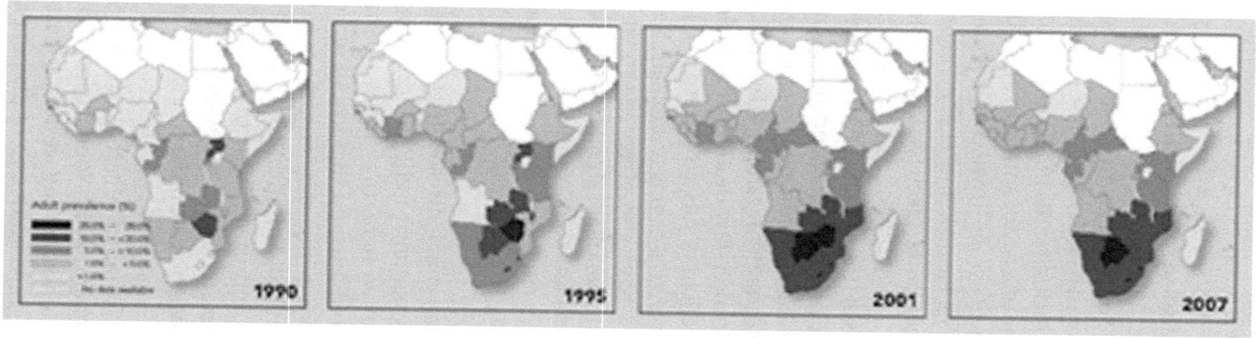

notable exceptions. Presidents Yoweri Museveni of Uganda and Abdou Diouf of Senegal are examples of African leaders who acted decisively in the early days of HIV/AIDS. More recently, governments like that of Botswana have also worked hard to contain HIV/AIDS and treat sufferers.

It is undoubtedly South Africa that has generated the most column inches with respect to HIV/AIDS. Former President Mbeki's 'dissident' views on HIV/AIDS, including his public questioning of the link between HIV and AIDS and the efficacy of antiretrovirals (ARVs) like AZT, achieved global notoriety. In 2000, he invited the prominent AIDS dissidents Peter Duesberg, David Rasnick and Harvey Bialy to serve on his Presidential AIDS Advisory Panel. Likewise, his Minister of Health, Dr Manto Tshabalala-Msimang (1999–2008) caused outrage by promoting beetroot, garlic and lemon juice as treatments for AIDS sufferers. While good policy-making may not have prevented the pandemic from spreading across South Africa, Mbeki and Tshabalala-Msimang's pronouncements undoubtedly intensified public uncertainty regarding HIV/AIDS and its spread. Furthermore, thousands of unnecessary deaths can be linked to the government's unpardonably slow rollout of ARVs (Nattrass 2007).

Mbeki was not, however, a complete anomaly. The views of other African leaders on HIV/AIDS have also given rise to concern. Speaking at the 88th Session of the International Labour Organization Conference in 2000, President Sam Nujoma (2000) of Namibia outlined his view of HIV/AIDS as a biological weapon and called on its disseminators to accept financial liability for combating it:

> HIV/AIDS is a man-made disease. It is not natural. States that produced chemical weapons to kill other nations are known, they are probably represented here, they know themselves too. We do not blame anybody but I would like to call upon employers, workers, governments, along with politicians whose parties are in opposition, non-governmental organisations represented here as well as those not represented, and the citizens of the world to unite as one and for those who created chemical weapons to kill other people, to make resources available in order to combat this scourge.

The declaration by Wangari Maathai, the Kenyan environmentalist, government minister and 2004 Nobel Peace prize-winner, that HIV was created as a biological weapon by western scientists to 'wipe out blacks' likewise created a significant degree of disquiet amongst AIDS activists (cited in the *Mail and Guardian* 18/10/2004).

Too much or too little? International responses

In 2007, an article in the *British Medical Journal* asking 'Are we spending too much on HIV?' ignited a long-smouldering debate over containment strategies. The author, Roger England (2007), asked whether, by treating HIV/AIDS as a 'special case', donors were ignoring other less media-prominent diseases – and healthcare infrastructure generally. England argued that celebrity endorsements have made funding HIV/ AIDS management 'fashionable'. Critics like England fear that HIV/AIDS has now become a *cause célèbre* and that, as a result, it is consuming a disproportionate degree of healthcare funding. HIV/AIDS will soon be absorbing nearly half of all donor aid for healthcare (OECD 2009, 2010) – a figure inconsistent, in the view of England and others like him, with the severity of its impact.

However, while HIV/AIDS may secure the lion's share of global healthcare funding, the fact remains that it is still under-resourced. Data from UNAIDS (2007) suggests a growing gap between 'resource needs and resource availability': $8.1 billion for 2007. Arguably, then, there is a case for increased levels of funding for healthcare across regions like sub-Saharan Africa. At the same time, the global economic downturn that began in 2007, and expensive military ventures like those conducted by the US and its allies in Afghanistan and Iraq, have put the squeeze on donor budgets, with Barack Obama announcing a freeze on US funding levels for HIV/AIDS (Zwillich 2009).

How much developed countries should contribute to combating HIV/ AIDS and how this aid should be disbursed is an important element of consideration for policymakers and aid workers alike. Under George W Bush, the US led the way in prioritizing funding for HIV/AIDS. The President's Emergency Plan for AIDS Relief (PEPFAR), reauthorized in 2008 with a budget of $48 billion, set the benchmark for other developed countries to follow. Under Bush, PEPFAR was controversial. It insisted on abstinence education as a prevention strategy, favoured faith-based organizations over secular NGOs, and became embroiled in debates regarding the use of generic drugs. Despite such issues, some of which may have been overemphasized or may with some justification be considered to have been 'teething pains', PEPFAR made HIV/AIDS a development priority for the US. However, one indisputable criticism is the fact that PEPFAR is bound by an unapologetically unilateral, top-down agenda. This puts it at odds with prevailing development trends, epitomized by the Global Fund and MAP, which stress the importance of multilateralism and partnership.

Gender and HIV/AIDS

A notable feature of the African AIDS pandemic is the disproportionate extent to which women are affected. The WHO (2003) has estimated that 58 percent of those infected with HIV in sub-Saharan Africa are women. However, even this figure underplays the severity of the gender imbalance. The gulf is especially wide when considering the 15 to 24 age group, where prevalence rates amongst young women far outstrip those of their male counterparts. While the disparity can be explained in part by physiological differences, the fact remains that young African women are one of the key 'at risk' groups. There are a number of possible explanations for this discrepancy, all of which are potentially controversial and emotive. Sexual violence in countries like Burundi, Central African Republic, the Democratic Republic of Congo, Liberia, Rwanda, Sierra Leone, South Africa and Sudan has, at times, reached unprecedented levels. (South Africa stands out from the other countries listed here because unlike them it is not a combat zone and it is neither currently destabilized nor a 'failed state'). Transactional sex is widespread across the continent. In addition, 'cultural' practices, including widow inheritance and widow 'cleansing', and high levels of intergenerational sex, all arguably contribute to women's powerlessness in determining their own sexual relationships. In July 2002, Stephen Lewis (2002), the then UN Secretary-General's Special Envoy on HIV/AIDS in Africa, described levels of HIV prevalence skewed by gender as presenting 'Africa and the world with a practical and moral challenge which places gender at the centre of the human condition. The practice of ignoring a gender analysis has turned out to be lethal'. Despite Rwanda and South Africa being ranked first and third (Inter-Parliamentary Union 2010) in the world respectively for their levels of female representation in parliament, gender hierarchies remain entrenched within these two countries and, indeed, across much of the continent. However, concentrating on gender hierarchies as a possible explanation for the rapid spread of HIV/AIDS has provoked a furious backlash from a number of quarters. Thabo Mbeki (2004) has claimed that such analysis is motivated by racism and aimed at portraying African men as promiscuous, diseased, misogynistic rapists. In a pamphlet distributed widely in South Africa, enigmatically entitled 'Castro Hlongwane, Caravans, Cats, Geese, Foot and Mouth and Statistics: HIV/AIDS and the Struggle for the Humanisation of the African', the anonymous author, generally believed to be Mbeki, argued that gender-based discourses effectively blame the victims by suggesting that HIV/AIDS is somehow 'self-inflicted'. The author refuted the perceived insinuation that '[African men] are prone to rape and abuse of women and that we uphold a value system that belongs to the world of wild animals, and that this accounts for the alleged "high incidence" of "HIV infection" in our country' (Anonymous 2002).

Regardless of the misgivings of Mbeki and others, the AIDS crisis in Africa has a clear gender dimension. All too frequently, violence against women and the spread of HIV/AIDS are dealt with as separate problems when in reality they are closely intertwined. Gender-based violence is often conceptualized within a human rights matrix and, in countries like South Africa, significant steps have been taken to ensure that men and women are equal before the law. The post-apartheid constitution is famously one of the most gender-liberal documents of its kind, enshrining as it does, by virtue of its 'Equality Clause', the rights of women in South African society. There is, however, a considerable gulf between legal niceties and the reality of South African women's experiences. In recent years, the pervasive and entrenched nature of violence against South African women has been laid bare in surveys such as the 2009 study in which 25 percent of male respondents admitted carrying out at least one rape (Jewkes *et al* 2009a). Whilst it is difficult to ascertain exact figures, incidences of rape in South Africa conceivably number in excess of half a million per year (SAPS 2005); evidence suggests that one third of South African women will be raped at some point in their lives (Moffett 2006). As the South African example highlights, that sub-Saharan African women are so disproportionately affected by HIV/AIDS is not 'just' a matter of biological susceptibility. It is the result of gross gender inequalities frequently made manifest in women's powerlessness over their own bodies.

Traditional medicine

If closer scrutiny of the uncomfortable subject of imbalanced gender hierarchies may help to explain the high prevalence rates of HIV/AIDS in Africa, then so too can analysis of indigenous representations of disease, indigenous knowledge systems and traditional medicine. It is said that up to 80 percent of people living in sub-Saharan Africa make regular use of the services of traditional healers (WHO 2002, 2008b). This is largely because the ratio of traditional healer to patient across the region generally varies between 1:200 and 1:400, while the ratio between that of medical doctor and patient frequently averages 1:20,000 (WHO 2002). Traditional healers, therefore, have a significant role to play where combating HIV/AIDS is concerned. However, from an HIV/AIDS perspective, there are a number of problems associated with the way in which disease is represented within many African cosmologies, and in the manner in which disease is diagnosed and treated. Once again, while it can be unhelpful to make gross generalizations about 'an African worldview', there is evidence to support the existence of what Ashforth (2001, 2002 and 2005) has termed a 'witchcraft paradigm' across much of the continent. Past and current anthropological and social studies document an African view of disease that is predicated on notions of witchcraft and sorcery (Evans-Pritchard 1937; Beattie 1963; Beidelman 1963; Buxton 1963; Ngubane 1977; Ingstad 1990; Meyer-Weitz *et al* 1998; Ashforth 2001, 2002, 2005; Niehaus 2001; Liddell *et al* 2005; Thomas 2008; Susser 2009).

At the heart of the 'witchcraft paradigm' is the idea that the only 'natural' death is that of old age; early death, debilitating illness and other misfortunes are all understood to occur as a result of witchcraft or supernatural forces such as those unleashed by displeased ancestors (Ashforth 2002; Ingstad 1990; Liddell *et al* 2005; Ngubane 1977). This cosmology renders the idea of a communicable pandemic like HIV/AIDS somewhat difficult to communicate and to comprehend. In most instances there are good reasons to celebrate diversity within belief systems. Critically, however, the witchcraft paradigm discourages the acceptance of random events as explanations for serious illness or death. The diagnosis of 'witchcraft' provides a 'rational' explanation for the 'unnaturalness' of an illness that causes people in their prime to waste away for no apparent reason. The bald reality is that the witchcraft paradigm detracts from the successful implementation of behavioural change and risk aversion strategies; according to this way of thinking, condoms cannot protect a person from witchcraft. Witchcraft is also understood to be victim-specific, as opposed to contagious. In terms of this way of thinking, a husband can place on his wife a charm that ensures that her illicit lovers contract specific STIs but that leaves him uninfected (Ngubane 1977). The ramifications of the promulgation of such a view are plain.

Traditional medicine is increasingly being taken seriously by health authorities. Both the World Health Organization (WHO 1976, 1990, 2002) and World Bank (2004) have produced strategies for incorporating and accommodating traditional medicines within broader healthcare systems. In some instances, the enhanced emphasis on traditional medicine is eminently practical; traditional remedies can be significantly cheaper than their biomedical equivalents.[4] However, traditional medicine's increasingly central role has also at times been politically motivated. In the interests of finding an 'African solution' to Africa's HIV/AIDS problem, the South African government engaged with a number of 'quack' scientists and dubious traditional healers. In particular, following Thabo Mbeki's climb-down over ARVs (Chapter 4), finding a 'traditional' alternative to ARVs became almost a matter of honour. Despite concerted efforts to prove otherwise, there is no clinical evidence to suggest that any traditional medicines, African or otherwise, are capable of treating AIDS (Pekala 2007). Some traditional remedies are in fact dangerous. Although accurate estimates are difficult to determine, evidence suggests that, in South Africa alone, traditional medicines used in the treatment of a variety of illnesses result in thousands of deaths per year (Popat *et al* 2001). Traditional medicinal compounds can include natural toxins such as *Euphorbia* (wartweed), *Solanum* (nightshade), *Datura* (Jamestown weed) and *Ricinis communis* (castorbean) as well as cantharides (Spanish fly) (Tagwireyi *et al* 2002). *Callilepis laureola* (ox-eye daisy), a herb common in Zulu herbal remedies, has been found to be extremely toxic, resulting in an estimated 1,500 deaths per year (Popat *et al* 2001). Metal salts, including copper sulphate and potassium dichromate, and other toxic substances such as potassium permanganate, paint thinners and turpentine, are also commonly used (Dunn *et al* 1991; Steenkamp *et al* 2002; Steenkamp 2002).

Obfuscation of the issues surrounding the efficacy and value of traditional medicines has led to a situation in which, in many instances, people infected with HIV believe such remedies to be part of a range of options available to them, often at the expense of the use of ARVs. While traditional healers, given their popularity and that their role within the structure of many African cosmologies affords them an important position in matters of healthcare, have a potentially-significant role within HIV/AIDS management, this should mainly be in the form of encouraging patients to be tested for HIV, to adhere to their prescribed ARV schedule and to employ risk aversion strategies in the interests of safeguarding themselves and their families.

Profiting from misery?

With respect to allopathic treatments, pharmaceutical companies have long been targeted as the villains of the HIV/AIDS story. The famous 2001 court case brought against the South African government by 39 pharmaceutical companies, over issues of copyright, licensing and the purchasing of generic drugs, is a case in point. The case, which was withdrawn before a ruling could be made, was an unmitigated public relations disaster for so-called 'Big Pharma' that brought its controversial role sharply into focus. At the heart of debates surrounding the position of the major drug companies is the goal of universal access to life-saving drugs versus the goal of patent protection. When the 1994 Trade Related Aspects of Intellectual Property Rights (TRIPS) agreement that forms part of the WTO framework was agreed, critics feared that the agreement would have a negative effect on drug provision in poorer countries. The basis for such concerns was that TRIPS, which dictates the intellectual property laws of the 153 WTO member states, would maintain high drug prices by undermining severely the viability of the generic pharmaceutical sector in countries like India. Given that ARV coverage in sub-Saharan Africa is approximately 44 percent (WHO 2009g), albeit up from an estimated 2 percent in 2003 (WHO 2008a), there is a clear argument for encouraging any strategy that makes such medicines more affordable. Apologists for the TRIPS regime are at pains to stress that the agreement does not offer blanket protection for the drug companies and that 'flexibilities' have been built into the system, allowing for compulsory licensing in the face of public health crises. However, few developing countries have sought to make full use of these flexibilities due, largely, to pressure from both the major pharmaceutical companies and the US government. The pharmaceutical companies argue that the debate concerning profits has been oversimplified and distorted, and that the research and development phase of bringing a drug to market is both expensive and time-consuming: $800 million and between ten and 15 years (PhRMA 2007). They claim that, without the possibility of recouping their investment, innovation will cease and the prospects for improved medicines and a vaccine or cure for HIV/AIDS will come to nothing. It is also possible to argue that there are far greater profits to be made investing in 'First World' afflictions such as high blood pressure, high cholesterol and heart disease. If pharmaceutical companies are not incentivized to invest in 'Third World' diseases, they may withdraw from this area of research.

At the same time, the fact remains that the mass production of generic ARVs has resulted in an almost inconceivable fall in the price of medicines used to treat HIV/AIDS, from approximately $10,000 a year during the mid-1990s to just over $100 per year in 2007 (WHO 2007a). A corresponding upsurge in coverage is also apparent. In 2003, ARV coverage in sub-Saharan Africa was just 2 percent; by 2007, this figure had risen to 30 percent (WHO 2008a). This was possible because the so-called 'first-line' therapies were developed during the 1990s, at a time before countries like India were fully TRIPS-compliant. The result was that, under Indian law, generic drug companies were able to 'reverse-engineer' first-line therapies and produce their own facsimiles. The patents for the new generation of more sophisticated, less toxic HIV/AIDS drugs, the 'second-line' therapies, are better protected by the TRIPS regime. This is deeply problematic. Patients gradually build up resistance to first-line therapies and eventually need to be moved onto new drug regimes. However, second-line therapies are between eight and 12 times more expensive than their first-line counterparts and, unless the prices of the former fall dramatically, potentially millions of people may be denied access to life-saving treatments (MSF 2009).

The determination of the pharmaceutical companies to protect their investments is evident from the sector's heavy lobbying of the US government and associated influence in shaping American policy on intellectual property rights. The stalled WTO negotiations have opened up increased opportunities for bilateralism, with the US negotiating free trade agreements with a number of countries/regions. In terms of protection for intellectual property, these agreements are usually 'TRIPS-plus' in that they tie partner countries to a regime that is more stringent still than that demanded by the WTO. Where countries like Brazil and Thailand have sought to maximize the advantages to be gained from the existing flexibilities inherent in TRIPS, they have come under sustained pressure from both pharmaceutical companies and the US government to desist. The result is that there is a considerable fear that second-line therapies may remain out of the reach of the majority of HIV/AIDS sufferers for years to come.

The politics of prevention

Preventing the spread of HIV/AIDS is as important as treating it; prevention is always better than cure. While this should represent a relatively uncontroversial starting point, the nature of HIV/AIDS prevention programmes has generated a significant degree of debate. Critically, the dialogue has been shaped profoundly by both internal and external actors, including the US government, the Catholic Church and other faith groups, and local political elites.

In developed countries, where HIV/AIDS has tended to affect 'risk populations' like homosexual men and sex workers, risk-reduction strategies such as encouraging increased condom usage have served to slow the pace of the epidemic. However, 'safer sex' messages have arguably been less successful in sub-Saharan Africa. There are many possible explanations for this. Both a lack of condom availability and cultural norms and values pertaining to fertility and sex can account for the relative lack of condom use across the continent. Faith-based groups like the Catholic Church and religiously-motivated politicians like former US President George W Bush and Ugandan President Yoweri Museveni have pressed instead for a 'social vaccine' based on abstinence for the young and fidelity for those in relationships. Uganda, with its dramatic fall in prevalence rates over the course of the 1990s, is held up as an alternative template to that offered by the proponents of 'safer sex'. President Museveni (2008) has claimed that the 'Ugandan miracle' of declining HIV prevalence was achieved largely without recourse to condoms and that his government's success lay in persuading teenagers to delay sexual debut and curb sexual excess.

There is no doubt that, given that Uganda is one of the few African success stories in the fight against HIV/AIDS, the potential value of transposing the 'Ugandan model' should be afforded significant consideration – but consideration must include rigorous analysis of the existing data, much of which currently remains open to interpretation. In many respects, the 'Ugandan model' continues to form the basis for ideological battles between those advocating a 'safer sex' approach to HIV prevention and those promoting instead a 'social vaccine'. Secular critics have campaigned vigorously against the 'ideological' nature of abstinence programmes, arguing that there is little evidence from, for example, the US to suggest that they actually succeed in delaying sexual debut. However, high-ranking Catholic officials, including the Pope (*The Lancet* 2009), the head of the Pontifical Council for the Family (1996) and the Bishop of Mozambique (*Guardian* 27/09/2007), have publicly questioned the use and value of condoms as a means of preventing HIV/AIDS. While in power, George W Bush (2004) was an ardent supporter of abstinence programmes, famously declaring that abstinence is 'the only 100 percent effective means of preventing pregnancy, HIV, and sexually-transmitted infections'. Under his administration, PEPFAR, in its original manifestation, dictated that 30 percent of all monies spent on prevention initiatives had to be targeted at abstinence programmes. Barack Obama has stated that US policy will henceforth be driven by 'best practice, not ideology', but abstinence education nonetheless remains an important element of the PEPFAR vision (cited in Walker 2009).

The politics and governance of HIV/AIDS

HIV/AIDS in Sub-Saharan Africa: Politics, Aid and Globalization brings together a number of elements that are relevant to those with interests in African Politics and History, Economics, Development, International Relations, Globalization and Gender Studies. While it is important to avoid the implication that the experience of the HIV/AIDS pandemic is uniform across the developing world in general, and across sub-Saharan Africa in particular, HIV/AIDS is, now more than ever, a disease that affects most adversely the poorest of those infected. It is increasingly a 'manageable condition' in developed countries, but a 'death sentence' in many poorer ones. International responses to HIV/AIDS in Africa highlight debates concerning unilateral versus multilateral approaches, with all the post-imperial baggage implied by this. In effect, HIV/AIDS epitomizes many components of North-South relations: questionable governance, underdevelopment, neo-imperialism and its resistance, and the contested nature of globalization.

1
Sex and Disease: A Historical Perspective

There is a scene in the film *Blood Diamond* (2006) in which Leonardo DiCaprio's character, Danny Archer, attempts to explain the roots of the 'African Crisis' to a newly-arrived American journalist played by Jennifer Connelly. Archer sums up the situation with a pithy acronym, 'TIA' – 'this is Africa'. The implication is that Africa is somehow both unknowable and inexplicable; a continent in which the normal 'rules' do not apply. It is due to the pernicious spread of this view across much of the developed world that a degree of ennui has crept into people's perceptions of the HIV/AIDS pandemic in Africa. HIV/AIDS is often treated as though it is without precedent, that it is unique in terms of African development; a disease lying outside the realms of historical context. There has also been an increased tendency on the part of policymakers to identify what makes Africa, and Africans, 'different' where HIV/AIDS is concerned. This chapter will address these trends, locate the disease within the broader 'African Crisis' and place HIV/AIDS within an appropriate historical context.

Perceptions of Africa, and of the 'African Crisis' generally, have long been coloured by the notion of a 'sick' continent. This viewpoint has continued, largely unbroken, from the early days of European intervention through to the current HIV/AIDS crisis. African explorers like David Livingstone regaled Europe with tales of exotic diseases and deadly parasites. Writing to a friend from Kuruman, in what is now the Northern Cape Province of South Africa, in 1841, Livingstone expressed his surprise at the poor health of local people, exclaiming that the 'Bechuanas have a great deal more disease than I expected to find among a savage nation' (Blaikie 2009). As imperial expansion intensified, West Africa came to be referred to by Europeans as the 'white man's grave'. Contemporary evidence tends to reinforce the stereotype of the 'sick continent'. Data from the United Nations makes it clear that Africa is once again lagging significantly behind the rest of the world where fundamental healthcare indicators are concerned. In basic terms, average life expectancy in sub-Saharan Africa rose from approximately 30 years just over a century ago to more than 50 by the early 1990s (cited in Adetunji and Bos 2006). However, HIV/AIDS has served to check this improvement and the consequences have been stark. In 2005, life expectancy for sub-Saharan Africans stood at 45.9 years, as opposed to an average of 67.3 years in Asia, the second-worst performing region. Meanwhile, in contrast, average life expectancy for Europeans stood at 73.7 years in 2005, nearly 40 percent higher than the figure for Africans (Adetunji and Bos 2006). The UNDP (2006) has estimated that, in some parts of Africa, HIV/AIDS curtails average life expectancy by almost 20 years. Healthcare indicators do not merely show that Africa is being left behind; they actually demonstrate a downward trend. Perhaps even more significantly, little has changed over the course of the past century to offset the grounds which exacerbated the spread of disease in the first place: in many respects, as will be demonstrated, debates past and present over healthcare in sub-Saharan Africa can be reduced to issues of infrastructure and access. However, this salient point has often been veiled (and continues to be veiled) by the tendency of the West to view Africans as somehow definable by their 'otherness'; their situation less the result of a lack of the medical infrastructure that will alleviate communicable disease in the way that it has been alleviated in richer countries and more the result of Africa being a place – and a set of circumstances – apart.

Africa's lack of healthcare infrastructure

Maureen Malowany (2000) argues that, if the history of epidemics in Africa has taught us anything, it is that the creation and maintenance of healthcare infrastructures is the key to combating HIV/AIDS. The evidence certainly stacks up in favour of this viewpoint. Sick people in Africa stand less chance of being adequately treated, for both communicable and non-communicable diseases, than those in any other region of the world. Africans therefore suffer higher rates of mortality when they fall ill. Healthcare is, as it has been since the colonial period, a matter for prioritized funding for donor agencies and fundraisers. However, if medical care were more readily available, then basic health indicators would rise accordingly. According to the WHO's 2006 Annual Report, 36 African countries have a shortage of trained medical personnel (WHO 2006a). The WHO (2006a) puts the total of full-time paid health workers (doctors, midwives and nurses) and support staff (pharmacists, technicians and clerical staff) worldwide at nearly 60 million, of whom just over 1.6 million are located in Africa. This is in comparison to Europe's total health workforce of 16 million workers and the Americas' 21 million. In terms of these estimates, the shortfall in the African health workforce is a minimum of 1.5 million personnel. In basic care terms, the ratio of doctor to patient in developed countries is approximately 1:500, while in African countries it is often under 1:25,000. The fact that up to 80 percent of people living in Africa consult traditional healers is testimony not only to the cultural importance of such healers but to the paucity of biomedical alternatives (see Chapter 5).

African doctor-patient ratios belie considerable imbalances between urban and rural areas. In Mozambique, 70 percent of doctors are located in Maputo, the capital (Shinn 2008). Where countries have created the capacity to train personnel, this advantage is often lost through excessive 'brain drain'. In this respect, Nigeria and South Africa are good examples. South Africa loses up to half of its medical graduates to developed countries each year. Similarly, over 21,000 Nigerian doctors are registered to practise in the US (Shinn 2008). The brain drain is reflected in the composition of healthcare professionals in the countries of the EU, the US and Canada; in Britain 33 percent of doctors were trained abroad, in the US, 27 percent and in Canada, 23 percent (WHO 2006a). The result is that Africa, with 24 percent of the global burden of disease, employs just 3 percent of the world's healthcare workers (WHO 2006a). If all the doctors trained in sub-Saharan Africa but currently working in OECD countries returned 'home', the number of doctors available would increase by 23 percent. In terms of basic healthcare infrastructure, too, sub-Saharan Africa fares badly. By the early 1990s, it was already apparent that HIV/AIDS could easily tip healthcare capacity beyond breaking point. Globally, African countries have the lowest proportion of hospital beds to population, with shortages exacerbated yet further in rural areas (Cabral 1993). The bald statistics highlighting this divide are that, according to the WHO (2009c), there are 79 hospital beds per 10,000 of population in Europe compared to less than ten beds per 10,000 of population in Africa. These issues are compounded by the fact that only two African countries, Botswana and The Gambia, have reached the 2001 Abuja Declaration target of allocating 15 percent of total government expenditure to health (African Union 2007). The lack of infrastructure means that Africa remains trapped in a medical age from which much of the world has moved on, in which communicable disease (alongside childbirth and perinatal conditions) poses the biggest threat to human health.

Communicable diseases become diseases of poverty

Communicable disease forms an important, albeit relatively little-discussed, part of the wider narrative of human history. It is disease, more than almost any other factor, which has shaped contemporary society. The Black Death caused fatalities on a scale that halved the medieval European population and undermined the feudal economic structure (Frank 1999). Likewise, the history of the Americas might have been very different if smallpox had not crippled the Aztec Empire, reducing the population of Central America from approximately 25 million in 1520 to just 700,000 within a century (Cook and Borah in Mann 2005). Would European domination of the 'New World' have been possible if existing American populations had not been reduced by up to 97 percent by the introduction of 'Old World' germs? Smallpox, measles, influenza, mumps, diphtheria and yellow fever have all cut a swathe through history (Crosby 2004). Yet, while history remembers great generals like Alexander the Great, Hannibal and Julius Caesar, together with the epic battles of antiquity – Thermopylae, Marathon, Issus and Cannae – it is frequently forgotten that disease often played a significant or determining role in war; an outbreak of plague arguably cost Athens the Peloponnesian War against Sparta, with over a third of the city's population succumbing to the epidemic in 430 BCE (Fox 2006). From time immemorial, disease, rather than the enemy, has tended to be the cause of most combatant deaths; dysentery and plague have long followed in the wake of armies on the move. That England's great warrior king, Henry V, died of dysentery rather than on the battlefield is indicative of the realities of medieval army life, as is the fact that at Agincourt in 1415, the scene of Henry's greatest triumph, dysentery affected his troops to the extent that many went into battle against the French naked from the waist down (Barker 2006). In terms of civilian casualties, millions more lost their lives to the Spanish influenza epidemic of 1918, which killed upwards of 50 million people worldwide, than died in theatre during World War I (Taubenberger and Morens 2006).

However, post-World War II, the global epidemiology of disease has changed quite remarkably. In the past, disease was capable of affecting rich and poor indiscriminately – smallpox killed Mary of Orange, Queen of England, Tsar Peter II of Russia and King Louis XV of France. Increasingly, however, communicable diseases have become overwhelmingly diseases of the poor. In developed countries, non-communicable diseases are now the major cause of death. Heart disease, strokes, cancer, diabetes and Alzheimer's disease are the five biggest killers in the US (CDC 2009).

In the EU, almost two-thirds of deaths are caused by heart disease or cancer (EPHA 2006). In contrast, the five leading causes of death in sub-Saharan Africa are HIV/AIDS, malaria, lower respiratory infections, diarrhoeal diseases, and perinatal conditions (WHO 2006a). Overall, in Africa, 72 percent of deaths are caused by communicable disease and complications arising from pregnancy and childbirth (WHO 2006b). The comparable figure from all other WHO regions combined stands at just 27 percent of fatalities. Never before has the dividing line between rich and poor been so stark.

Africa's reputation as the 'sick continent' of the world is not unfounded. Based on UN figures, it is clear that, in terms of basic indicators like life expectancy, sub-Saharan African has progressed very little in the past five decades (see Table 1.1). While other developing regions – Asia and South America – have demonstrated significant gains, with life expectancy in Asia climbing by almost 20 years between 1960 and 2004, African progression stalled in the late 1980s/early 1990s and subsequently went into reverse. Other indicators tend to convey a similar message. The global Human Development Index, calculated according to indicators including life expectancy, adult literacy figures and per capita income, places African states as 24 of the 25 worst-performing countries (see Table 1.2). Whereas epidemic-type diseases largely disappeared from developed regions early in the twentieth century, African history is replete with examples that have killed, and often continue to kill, millions: smallpox, malaria, tuberculosis, sleeping sickness, yellow fever, syphilis, and, most recently, HIV/AIDS. That the continent remains mired in the sicknesses of another age is evidenced by the fact that in Africa infectious diseases account for nearly 70 percent of the disease burden. In Europe, they account for less than 20 percent (WHO 2000). Historically, the majority of biomedical campaigners have tended to consider Africa as a 'special case' where each

Table 1.1   Life Expectancy at Birth for World and UN Regions, 1960–2005

Region	1960–69	1970–79	1980–89	1990–99	2000–04
World	52.5	58.1	61.4	63.7	65.4
Sub-Saharan Africa	42.4	46.3	49.0	47.6	45.9
Asia	48.5	56.4	60.4	64.0	67.3
Europe	69.6	71.0	72.0	72.6	73.7
Latin America and Caribbean	56.8	60.9	64.9	68.3	71.5
Northern America	70.1	71.6	74.3	75.5	77.6
Oceania	63.7	65.8	69.3	71.5	74.0

Table 1.2   Human Development Index (179 Countries)

Countries demonstrating 'High Human Development' in order of Rank	Countries Demonstrating 'Low Human Development' in order of Rank
1 Iceland	170 Chad
2 Norway	171 Guinea-Bissau
3 Canada	172 Burundi
4 Australia	173 Burkina Faso
5 Ireland	174 Niger
6 Netherlands	175 Mozambique
7 Sweden	176 Liberia
8 Japan	177 Democratic Republic of the Congo
9 Luxembourg	178 Central African Republic
10 Switzerland	179 Sierra Leone

Source: (UNDP 2008)

of the above diseases has been concerned; there has been a tendency to view the African incidence of HIV/AIDS in the same way.

Communicable disease, paternalism and control

The former President of South Africa, Thabo Mbeki (2004), has argued that much of the HIV/AIDS discourse is racist, since a significant degree of the material linked to the pandemic seeks, in his view, to blame the victim for his or her infection. Mbeki has emphasized the subjectivity of the current presupposition that only Western medicine and Western science are capable of 'saving' Africa from itself. In this particular argument, history is on his side. The discourse of disease and healing in Africa has, even from before the earliest days of the 'scramble' for Africa, been tinged with the paternalism of imperial and colonial bureaucrats, medical practitioners and missionaries. Medical studies celebrated the victories of Western biomedicine, medical science and technology over African disease. Texts like Michael Gelfand's (1953) *Tropical Victory: An Account of the Influence of Medicine on the History of Southern Rhodesia* (now Zimbabwe) gloried in the role played by biomedicine in improving life expectancy in southern Africa. Gelfand's approach is, on the one hand, entirely justifiable. On the other hand, however, it is difficult to disassociate the positive changes noted by him from the insidious top-down perspective that continually reinforced the notion of 'active' Europe as the saviour of 'passive' Africa – and the associated rationalization of colonial control. The high incidence of human trypanosomiasis, or sleeping sickness, yellow fever, bilharzia and rinderpest (cattle plague) in the early decades of the twentieth century fascinated colonial authorities, who set about endeavouring to 'conquer' disease in Africa. How to understand and manage epidemics became a central tenet of the colonial overseer's armoury (Malowany 2000). Many of these colonial-era diseases, in particular sleeping sickness and its pernicious spread, came to obsess administrators across much of sub-Saharan Africa. Sleeping sickness was linked quickly to human migration which, in turn, gave the authorities in, for instance, the Belgian Congo the excuse to impose further social controls on subject populations (Malowany 2000). As with HIV/AIDS and much of sub-Saharan Africa nearly a century later, public health in the Belgian Congo became synonymous with sleeping sickness during the early twentieth century (Beinart and Hughes 2007). By the mid-1960s, assiduous campaigns effectively eradicated the disease from most of the continent. It has subsequently resurfaced, largely due to the breakdown in health sector governance that follows civil conflict and the mass migration of refugees. There are currently 60 million people at risk from sleeping sickness in 36 countries in sub-Saharan Africa, the majority of them in the DRC (MSF 2010). The 1950s and 1960s also saw concerted campaigns to eradicate smallpox and malaria. As a result, by the early 1980s, smallpox was virtually eliminated. For a number of reasons, the campaigns against malaria have been less successful: the costs associated with the widespread application of insecticides such as DDT, concerns regarding the environmental and health effects of DDT and related programmes, and the growing insecticide-resistance of mosquitoes in certain areas (Sweeney 1999).

The attitudes of colonial elites towards the people living under their jurisdiction were by no means homogenous. In their control of subject peoples, different European powers exhibited different agendas and methods. Critically, however, a fixation with sexuality, morality and disease figured strongly in the rationalization of most European rule in Africa. Accordingly, much of the relevant language within colonial and imperial discourse is dehumanizing and prurient. Since the idea of 'progress' lay at the heart of the Victorian mindset, a fear of 'degenerative elements' that might impede that progress obsessed the burgeoning middle class that formed the bedrock of colonial and imperial expansion (McClintock 1995). Critically, elites' linkage of 'degenerative elements' with 'the other' provided the former with corresponding evidence of their own ostensible 'progression'. Much of this mindset was modelled on a form of social Darwinism that embraced the emergent 'racial sciences' of eugenics and craniometry. These pseudo-sciences re-enforced views of racial superiority and dovetailed well with European perceptions of a hierarchical 'natural order' of humanity. Disease and contagion were associated obsessions that enabled Victorian policymakers to justify their imposition of 'discipline' on all elements that might potentially counteract the mental and physical wellbeing of a given society. Sex and health increasingly came to be seen as being linked inextricably (Lyons and Lyons 2004). In the metropoles – especially Britain – this meant keeping the 'baser instincts' of the working classes, and especially working-class women, in check. In the colonies, it resulted in similar attempts to control (and, as colonial administrators saw it, 'improve') colonized societies (McClintock 1995). Women in particular were viewed as potential sources of 'contagion' and elites became increasingly fixated with the management of women's sexuality, both at home and abroad. The result was that by the end of the nineteenth century Europeans had come to view sexual 'purity' as a defining characteristic of an 'advanced' society. Colonial discourses on African sexuality provided European elites with further 'proof' of white racial superiority (Cooper and Stoler 1989). According to Birkbeck historian Daniel Pick's (1993) *Faces of Degeneration: A European Disorder*:

> social Darwinism and other evolutionary theories in the later-nineteenth century underpinned the supremacist rhetoric but the spectre of internal degeneration continually haunted it.

In settled colonial societies like South Africa, control of sexual behaviour and 'morality' therefore formed one of the key planks of a worldview geared towards safeguarding European privilege through emphasis on the African 'other' (Stemmet 2003).

Where culture, sexuality and disease were concerned, hypocrisy and double standards were part and parcel of the narrative of imperial expansion, a narrative that has, moreover, proved remarkably durable. In this respect, Thabo Mbeki's (2004) observation that the people of Africa are habitually viewed by outsiders as 'diseased, corrupt, violent, amoral [and] sexually depraved' has struck a chord across the continent.

The discourse of sex and disease in Africa

'Anthropological' discussions of sexuality often say more about the observer than the observed. Much about Western sexuality can be read into the frequently salacious and even pornographic nature of colonial anthropological and ethnographical literature. There is no doubt that narratives of African sexuality have been employed time and again to buttress Western conceptions of morality (Lyons and Lyons 2004), and it is therefore tempting to avoid adding to the historiography. However, given the frequency with which debates on sexual 'morality' occur when HIV/AIDS is discussed and related policy formulated, it is important to engage, at least to some extent, with the relevant discourses.

HIV/AIDS is only the most recent of a number of sexually-transmitted diseases that have been viewed as threatening the African continent with 'extinction'. In seeking to provide a rationale for the depth and scope of these diseases, analysts have regularly emphasized issues of culture – particularly sexual norms – above issues of healthcare infrastructure. In the early days of HIV/AIDS, researchers had to confront the differences between the African experience and the European and North American experience. They sought to understand and explain why a disease that in the developed world was spreading primarily through high-risk groups of homosexual men and intravenous drug users was now rampaging through heterosexual populations across significant stretches of sub-Saharan Africa. As in the past, conceptions of African sexuality became a key area of consideration.

The idea that African sexuality was somehow unusually uncontrolled and immoderate was a view commonly held by Europeans during the colonial era (Vaughan 1991). Reacting to a 1920 study by Edwin Smith and Andrew Dale of the Ila-speaking communities of Northern Rhodesia's Namwala District, a reviewer in the *Journal of the African Society* felt moved to comment that 'no European can be long in contact with Bantu people without realising the important part played in their lives by sexual matters' (McI. [*sic*] 1921). In the Ila study, Smith and Dale expressed a horror of 'the unproductiveness caused by the astonishing promiscuity of their sexual relations and the extreme earliness of age at which these relations commence. It is no exaggeration to state that from the age of seven or eight a girl, married or otherwise, counts her lovers, who are constantly changing' (Smith and Dale 2003). Countless similar examples abound in the literature. In a 1926 article in *Africa* discussing 'the principles of Bantu marriage', the author warns that rampant promiscuity is reported from every corner of 'Bantuland' (Torday 1929). A prurient fascination with sexual mores is apparent; the European view of African sexuality was from the outset framed as an aspect of the 'other':

The few examples which will be quoted are fair specimens of what we hear from other quarters. Bangala girls have free ingress from an early age to *mbongi*, the house of bachelors. Among the Warega sexual intercourse is practised between unmarried people of different sexes before puberty. 'Several tribes permit sexual intercourse between immature children and regard it in the light of play.' Among the Basonge, sexual intercourse takes place between children a considerable time before puberty. No Herero girl is a virgin when she comes to the initiation ceremony. The utmost liberty is left to unmarried Matabele girls. Even before puberty Luba boys and girls arrange secret meetings in the bush and on the river bank. It can serve little purpose to extend this list. Some of the most competent philologists assure us that in most Bantu languages there is no word for 'virgin' (Torday 1929).

Much of the above is replicated within contemporary HIV/AIDS discourse, where there is a still-prurient fascination with exploring 'African' sexual practices, often in conjunction with the determination of accompanying levels of promiscuity (Nguyen and Stovel 2004). However, there have also been meaningful, albeit problematic, attempts to identify cultural inducements to risk. A much-cited study by Caldwell *et al* (1989), which outlined the possibility of a 'distinct African sexual system', brought cultural explanations for the spread of HIV/AIDS in sub-Saharan Africa to the fore. The authors argued that acknowledging socio-cultural differences in the construction of sexuality in different regions was crucial to developing a deeper understanding of the emergent African pandemic. Writing in the late 1980s, the authors argued that 'there is a distinct and internally coherent African system embracing sexuality, marriage, and much else ... it is no more right or wrong, progressive or unprogressive than the Western system' (Caldwell *et al* 1989). It was argued that, because African societies place a high value on fertility, 'virtue is related more to success in reproduction than to limiting profligacy' (Caldwell *et al* 1989). Caldwell *et al* also argued that polygamy, the intergenerational nature of most marriages, and certain sex taboos including post-partum abstinence encourage both formal and informal multiple partner relationships. They contended that, rather than making pejorative statements, they were simply highlighting that, unlike the more ostensibly puritanical European moral compass, sexual limitations do not lie at the centre of the African moral universe. Caldwell *et al* were not alone. Their argument was reinforced by a study by Odebiyi and Vivekananda (1991) that similarly pointed to the centrality of 'cultural features' to the spread of HIV/AIDS across sub-Saharan Africa. Caldwell *et al* (1989) linked the commonplace nature of open 'transactional sex' in Africa to the fact that it is culturally acceptable in a way that would bring opprobrium in the West. In a similar vein, it has also been argued that because fertility is so highly prized in many African societies it is common for women to have children prior to marriage in order to demonstrate their fertility (Meekersa and Calvès 1997). The net result, according to this view, is that Africans tend have multiple sexual partners and are therefore more susceptible to the spread of sexually-transmitted diseases.

However, critiques of the notion of a 'distinct African sexual system' as outlined above were quick to surface (Le Blanc *et al* 1991; Heald 1995). The work by Caldwell *et al* (1989) was criticized as being 'fraught with serious methodological flaws' (Le Blanc *et al* 1991) and for the 'value implications' inherent in the analysis (Heald 1995). In terms of methodology, the main flaws were held to be the lack of regional representation at the heart of the study, together with the dated surveys (conducted prior to the 1970s) on which the authors drew (Le Blanc *et al* 1991). Caldwell *et al* stood accused of extrapolating data from a small number of studies in order to present the 'totality' of the continent.

Incontestable, however, is the fact that, across much of sub-Saharan Africa, levels of sexually-transmitted diseases have been, and continue to be, disproportionately high. In 1981, just prior to the era of AIDS in Africa, Abimbola Osoba (1981) highlighted the pervasiveness of gonorrhoea and syphilis across tropical Africa. He suggested that gonorrhoea was widely prevalent within some communities, to the point that it was 'regarded as a sign of adolescence or sexual potency'. He emphasized how, in comparative terms, African prevalence rates for sexually-transmitted diseases far outstripped those of developed countries:

> When the prevalence rates of some African countries are compared with those of the developed countries, it is obvious that STDs in Africa constitute a major public health problem. For example, the rate for gonorrhoea per 100 000 population in Kampala (Uganda) is 10 000 and in Nairobi (Kenya) it is 7000; the corresponding figures for Greater London (Britain) and Atlanta (USA) are 310 and 2510 respectively (Osoba 1981).

With respect to syphilis, Osoba (1981) argued strongly that 'the prevalence is certainly considerably higher than in Europe and the USA and is totally unacceptable; it therefore demands concern and energetic control measures'. During the 1990s, there was little evidence to suggest an improvement. According to the WHO (1995), infection by trichomoniasis, chlamydia, syphilis and gonorrhoea affected 9 percent of Americans aged between 15 and 44 annually. The corresponding figure for sub-Saharan Africa was 25 percent. The 1995 WHO survey found that more than 40 percent of women attending prenatal clinics in Uganda and Botswana were infected with trichomoniasis (WHO 1995). Determination of causal factors aside, these figures are important because they demonstrate that HIV/AIDS is only one of a number of sexually-transmitted diseases still striking sub-Saharan Africa. They also reveal how these diseases have, in recent decades at least, affected Africa to a far greater extent than they have other regions. Finally, they form one additional piece of the African HIV/AIDS puzzle: epidemiological studies suggest that having a sexually-transmitted disease can increase an individual's chances of contracting HIV by up to 400 percent (WHO 1995).

A precursor to HIV/AIDS discourse: Syphilis in colonial Africa

Given their discoursal similarities, the African syphilis epidemics of the early- to mid-twentieth century provide a pertinent literary and historiographical precursor to the HIV/AIDS pandemic. Karen Jochelson's (1991) observation that the story of HIV could be encapsulated in the phrase 'old crisis, new virus' seems a prescient one. Shula Marks (2002) has argued that, with respect to South Africa, HIV/AIDS was an epidemic 'waiting to happen', pointing to the syphilis epidemic as an earlier product of a socio-economic system that made the rapid dissemination of a disease like HIV/AIDS almost inevitable. HIV/AIDS, particularly in the early days of the pandemic, was viewed globally as a disease introduced and spread by foreigners and/or 'degenerates' with its materialization being accompanied by warnings of moral collapse and social decline. Sexually-transmitted diseases have long been viewed in this way. The extent to which the proclivities and peccadilloes of 'other' nations and societies have been blamed for the introduction and dissemination of sexually-transmitted diseases into 'home' populations is enlightening. Throughout history, stigmatization of the 'other' has afforded victims of disease and their communities both an explanation for their suffering and a convenient scapegoat.

The debates surrounding the geographical origins of syphilis are contentious.[1] It has been argued widely that syphilis was a 'New World' disease introduced to Europe by sailors returning from the Americas in the 1490s (Barlow 2006; Bollet 2004; Crosby 2004). However, there are passages in the Bible that could conceivably describe syphilis. In Deuteronomy Chapter 28, Verse 27, those who failed to obey God's commands were threatened with the 'Botch of Egypt ... the emerods, and ... the scab, and ... the itch, whereof thou canst not be healed' (King James Version). Further passages in Job, Jeremiah and Numbers describe symptoms – genital lesions, failing eyesight, shooting pains in the joints, mucous patches, skin discolouration and depigmentation – that are all suggestive of syphilis (Baker *et al* 1988). Proponents of an 'Old World' origin contend that prior to the fifteenth century syphilis was relatively indistinguishable from leprosy (Baker *et al* 1988). If syphilis was indeed prevalent in Eurasia and Africa in the pre-Columbian era, then it existed in a relatively non-virulent form. At the end of the fifteenth century, it suddenly became recognizable as a separate disease.[2] The siege of Naples by Charles VIII of France in 1495 is said to have marked the onset of the 'age of syphilis' in Europe. As the story goes, Spanish mercenaries in Charles' army, who had sailed previously with Columbus and contracted syphilis from Amerindians, communicated their infection to Charles' camp. Almost from the outset, the national 'blame-game' began. The Neapolitans referred to syphilis as the 'French disease', Charles VIII called it the 'Neapolitan disease'. In France it was called the 'Spanish disease', while the Spanish knew it as the 'West Indian disease'. In India, where it is said to have arrived with Vasco da Gama in 1498, it was called the 'Portuguese sore' or the 'European illness' (Bollet 2004). In Africa, the pattern was no different. Zulus named it the 'disease of the white men' (Kark 2003). By the late nineteenth century, syphilis appears to have been relatively widespread across East Africa in general, and across Uganda in particular. The parallels between the Ugandan HIV/AIDS narrative (see Chapter 7) and the historiography of the assessment and containment of syphilis are noteworthy. The analysis of syphilis epidemics emanating from West Africa (Willcox 1946) and southern Africa (Kark 2003) is similarly pertinent.

In 1907, the British Foreign Office sent a venereal disease specialist from the Royal Army Medical Corps, Lieutenant-Colonel F. J. Lambkin, to investigate a Ugandan syphilis epidemic. Lambkin (1914), believing Uganda to have been 'virgin soil' where syphilis was concerned, concluded that it had been introduced into the area in the mid-nineteenth century by Arab traders. Whatever the veracity or otherwise of his ideas about origin, his incidence statistics for the colony were alarming. Certain districts, he claimed, had infection rates of up to 90 percent, with accompanying infant mortality standing at 50 to 60 percent. Overall, he believed at least half the population to be affected. In the 1930s, further Ugandan studies estimated that 60 percent of antenatal patients 'showed evidence of syphilis' (cited in Davies 1956). At the same time, evidence from other studies suggests a much lower incidence rate, perhaps as low as 11 percent. The disparity highlights the difficulties in tracing disease incidence in history. In this case, syphilis may have been confused with yaws (Davies 1956).

Overt notions of racial superiority make it particularly difficult to gauge correctly the veracity of pre-apartheid- and apartheid-era South African studies of disease. However, it appears that syphilis was largely unknown in South Africa until the late nineteenth century, by which time it had begun to spread rapidly (Jochelson 1999). Evidence suggests that it was widespread by the early decades of the twentieth century, but here an even more distinctly racist agenda clouds the narrative. A 1919 study published in the *South African Medical Record* estimated an infection rate of between 20 and 25 percent. However, its author, Dr A Pijper (1919), was at pains to point out that that none of the white South Africans in his sample were infected, and that, in his view, it was now effectively a black South African disease. Studies from West Africa also indicate a significant degree of infection from diseases including gonorrhoea and syphilis. Medical records from the British armed forces in the mid-1940s reported that 60 percent of Nigerian troops were infected with venereal disease, and that 50 percent of troops from the Gold Coast and 28 percent from Sierra Leone were similarly affected (Willcox 1946).

Clearly, there are links to be found between early non-African attempts to 'understand African sexual behaviour' and the direction taken by current HIV/AIDS debates. Disease incidence has been framed in a distinctly subjective manner; 'African culture' has itself come to be seen as a barrier to disease management – a debate that will be addressed in more detail in Chapter 5. By 1985, commentators were already blaming the heterosexual nature of HIV/AIDS in Africa on 'high levels of sexual promiscuity' (cited in Packard and Epstein 1991). Thabo Mbeki spoke for many Africans when he highlighted how HIV/AIDS discourse has emphasized problems with 'African sexuality' and 'African behaviour' over differences in socio-economic status between Africans and Europeans and North Americans. Rather than providing insight into the problem of HIV/AIDS itself, the trajectory of contemporary HIV/AIDS discourse speaks volumes about the prejudices, conscious or otherwise, of Western analysts. Again, there are historical precedents. The researchers engaged in the suppression of syphilis outbreaks in colonial Africa focused on why the disease affected African populations in the way that it did and why the African experience of the disease differed from Western experience (Packard and Epstein 1991).

At the same time, it is also possible to detect within some colonial discussions on syphilis evidence of embryonic debates concerning the role of gender hierarchies, migrant labour, social disintegration and risk behaviours, and the lack of public awareness about disease transmission, alongside an emergent understanding of how these factors might contribute to the evolution of disease epidemics (Davies 1956; Lambkin 1914; Kark 2003; Rampen 1978; Willcox 1946). In 1949, Sydney Kark's (2003) seminal article on 'The social pathology of syphilis in Africans', was published in the *South African Medical Journal*. Sixty years on, his essay makes remarkable reading, largely because if throughout the text 'syphilis' is substituted with 'HIV/AIDS', the piece would be all but indistinguishable from any number of contemporary articles on the latter. In a radical departure from the 'anthropological' focus of his apartheid and colonial peers, Kark (2003), who conducted the bulk of his research in South Africa during the 1930s and 1940s, put forward a socio-economic explanation for the spread of syphilis. The high incidence of syphilis was caused, he argued, neither by 'the nature of the African' nor 'primitive' social customs. Rather, it was the result of the collapse of social cohesion, brought about by the onset of the migrant labour system. Kark (2003) made the point that 'the problem of syphilis in South Africa is so closely related to the development of the country that a study of the social factors responsible for its spread is likely to assist in its control'. In much the same way, early epidemiological profiling attempted to identify the social factors lying at the heart of the HIV/AIDS pandemic – essentially, the 'specificities' of the African experience (Nguyen and Stovel 2004).

In recent years, the 'social pathology' of HIV/AIDS has been frequently discussed as though it is without precedent (Marks 2002). However, as Kark's work testifies, this is by no means the case. Kark cited the destruction of the fabric of traditional societies and the resultant disintegration of societal norms governing sexual behaviour as key factors in the rampant proliferation of syphilis across 1940s South Africa. He contended that migrant labour produced 'great changes in Bantu social customs, breaking down a system of rigid moral standards, destroying the old concepts of right and wrong, cheapening relations between men and women and bringing with it syphilis' (Kark 2003). He went on to argue that the 'first line of treatment must be to remedy the unhealthy social relationships' that had created the conditions in which the epidemic was able to develop. Even Kark's hypothesis, however, was not the first of its kind. Lambkin, the venereal disease specialist sent to Uganda, had reached a number of similar conclusions before WWI. He, too, pointed to the disintegration of social norms in the face of colonial intrusion as the cause of a collapse of the rules governing sexual behaviour. For Lambkin, the relative 'emancipation' of Bugandan women following the introduction of Christianity resulted in greater sexual promiscuity: '[the] abandonment of polygamy and the old restrictions on the liberty of the women [was] probably the chief cause of the outbreak' (Lambkin 1914). Anthony Zwi and Antonio Cabral (1991), writing before HIV/AIDS became a full-blown pandemic in South Africa, warned that 'high risk' situations likely to exacerbate the spread of the disease 'occur where there is diminished concern about health, increased risk taking, and reduced social concern about casual sexual rela-tionships'. Compare Zwi and Cabral's analysis to that of Kark (2003) half a century earlier, when he argued that 'the code of morals of the men who have been to town appears [to be] one that does not regard sexual intercourse in a serious light, but as a cheap commodity for temporary pleasure'.

There are other parallels between both the incidence and the analysis of syphilis and HIV/AIDS in sub-Saharan Africa. Both diseases have been associated with 'foreigners', disease-testing has been patchy, and treatment has been expensive and restricted (Heimer 2007). The story of HIV/AIDS in sub-Saharan Africa is therefore by no means new. Once contextualized, its rapid spread through much of the continent becomes increasingly comprehensible; in southern Africa, its emergence as a pandemic appears all but inevitable.

Conclusion

Where HIV/AIDS is concerned, much has been made of the question 'why Africa?' In this respect, contextualization is everything. To date, analysis has been hampered by ongoing efforts to reinvent the wheel. While the emergence of the disease itself might be relatively recent (Chapter 2), the history of illness in Africa reflects how the conditions that precipitated and facilitated its spread are by no means new. Karen Jochelson's summing-up of the African AIDS crisis as 'old crisis, new virus' could not be more prescient. Many of the issues that have been understood to be unique to the HIV/AIDS narrative have precedents in other epidemics. In particular, the African syphilis epidemics of the early twentieth century shed a significant amount of light on the social pathology of HIV/AIDS. Syphilis was associated with the 'extinction' of local populations. It was sexually transmitted, it provoked debates centred on questions of sexual morality and it reinforced Europeans' preconceived image of Africans as over-sexed and promiscuous. High prevalence rates of syphilis, together with other sexually-transmitted diseases, combined to buttress the outsider view that there was some-thing 'different' about African societies. During the colonial era, it was easy to lay the blame for syphilis on the victims themselves. As a sexually-transmitted disease, it could be viewed as a 'disease of choice'. In many respects, this predilection has been carried over into current outsider perceptions of victims of HIV/AIDS in Africa. In essence, the problem is seen to lie with Africans themselves; if 'they' would only change 'their' behaviour then the crisis would recede. At the same time it is possible to discern, within colonial disease narratives relating to southern Africa in particular, the dawning realization that the spread of syphilis was linked to the cataclysmic breakdown of societal norms and values engendered by the colonial-induced migrant labour system. Syphilis therefore sparked embryonic discussions on gender (Chapter 3) and the socio-political economy of the African state.

Effective HIV/AIDS management calls for cooperation at a global level. Arguably, as with any situation involving the emotive issues of culture and sexuality, the best way forward is for researchers and policymakers alike to 'work with, not on, African communities in order to facilitate their own informed management of sexual health' (Kesby *et al* 2003). The moral dimension inherent within the PEPFAR agenda, with its strong proscriptions on premarital sex and prostitution, may be counterproductive (Chapter 6 and Chapter 7). Contrary to sex-and-disease discourses – both historical and contemporary – that serve to focus attention on the 'otherness' of the African situation, evidence suggests that the solution to overcoming epidemics in Africa was, and remains, the establishment and maintenance of a robust healthcare infrastructure. Rather than pigeon-holing HIV/AIDS as a 'special issue' and funding it accordingly, its effective management should be considered to be one aspect – albeit an important one – of a prioritized African healthcare agenda (Chapter 6).

2
The Origins of HIV/AIDS

Why has Africa suffered so disproportionately from HIV/AIDS? This is the question at the heart of this study. One possible explanation relates to the origins of HIV, the virus that causes AIDS. The bald statistics bear repeating: by late 2008, an estimated 33.4 million people were infected with HIV/AIDS worldwide. Sufferers in sub-Saharan Africa made up two-thirds of this total (UNAIDS 2009a). That HIV originated in Africa is, conspiracy theories aside, undisputed. This being the case, it is hardly surprising that HIV/AIDS managed to gain a strong foothold on the continent. After all, HIV was not identified positively until 1983 and even then remained little understood for some years. A simple answer, therefore, to the question of 'why Africa?' is that Africa represents 'ground zero' (Iliffe 2006).

Our understanding of the origins and mechanics of HIV/AIDS developed relatively slowly. This allowed for the evolution of a burgeoning social narrative that reflected people's anxieties and prejudices about a frightening new disease. Confusion as to how HIV/AIDS was spread, the fact that it was fatal and that it appeared, in the early days of the pandemic, to prey on those frequently on the margins of mainstream society: homosexuals, drug addicts and sex workers, stigmatized sufferers in ways that continue to this day. In the past, therefore, African leaders have been understandably reluctant to accept an African origin for HIV/AIDS. However, the source of HIV/AIDS can now without doubt be traced to Western Equatorial Africa,[1] where the viral ancestors of HIV-1 and HIV-2[2] have been located in groups of chimpanzees and sooty mangabeys respectively (Sharp *et al* 2000). At the same time, exactly how these viral ancestors, the Simian Immunodeficiency Viruses (SIVs), made the 'leap' to HIV remains a hotly-contested debate. Explanations vary, ranging from bestiality to colonial inoculation programmes, with a great many other hypotheses in between. Diseases regularly 'jump' from animals to humans (smallpox, measles and influenza all originate from domesticated animals), but humans in West Equatorial Africa have been in contact with chimpanzees and sooty mangabeys for millennia, and the advent of HIV/AIDS is comparatively recent. For some (Pascal 1991; Hooper 1999), the onset of HIV/AIDS is 'man-made' and the pandemic is one aspect of the all-pervasive colonial legacy. Others have questioned the value of determining the exact causes of the jump. In the late 1980s, the head of the Ugandan AIDS Committee argued that combating HIV/AIDS should take priority over efforts to pinpoint its origins, commenting that 'there is a snake in the house. Do you just sit and ask where the snake came from?' (Rödlach 2006). Conversely, at a Royal Society meeting called to discuss the origins of HIV/AIDS, Kevin De Cock (2001) acknowledged that although 'the origins of HIV-1 and HIV-2 seem academic questions compared with the urgent needs for prevention and care, public health cannot ignore how the acquired immune deficiency syndrome (AIDS) pandemic emerged'. For countries closest to the epicentre, a 'ground zero' explanation for the rapid spread of HIV/AIDS across much of sub-Saharan Africa removes the charges of culpability for inaction, at least during the 1980s. For this reason alone, the origins of HIV/AIDS should be considered, although not in isolation from the wider story.

A new disease

As outlined in Chapter 1, major pandemics are not without historical precedent. Some, like the Black Death, linger in the public imagination for centuries, while others move to the margins of the collective consciousness. The influenza or 'Spanish Flu' epidemic of 1918–1920 that killed, depending on estimates, upwards of 40 million people in just over two years has been described by Alfred W. Crosby as a 'forgotten pandemic' (Crosby 2003). In terms of severity, the influenza strain that caused the 'forgotten pandemic' was far more virulent than HIV/AIDS. It is possible that some 500 million people worldwide – one-third of the global population at the time – might have been infected (Taubenberger and Morens 2006). Malaria, after HIV/AIDS the leading cause of death in sub-Saharan Africa, receives pitifully few headlines. HIV/AIDS' continuing influence on the global consciousness is evidence that it, like the Black Death, is seen as a disease 'apart'. This is due, at least in part, to its origins and means of transmission.

As 'Acquired Immunodeficiency Syndrome' suggests, AIDS is not a specific disease *per se*. AIDS is brought on by the Human Immunodeficiency
Virus (HIV), a retrovirus[3] that attacks the body's immune system over
a number of years. HIV breaks down slowly an individual's ability to
ward off opportunistic infections including pneumocystis pneumonia
and mycobacterial (bacteria that can cause tuberculosis and leprosy),
cryptococcal and toxoplasmic (which can cause meningitis and encephalitis respectively) diseases. HIV also leaves the body highly vulnerable
to certain cancers, including Kaposi's sarcoma and lymphoma. Death
from AIDS comes as a result of the onset of any number of these infections and diseases, against which, once the immune system has collapsed,
the body has little defence (Whiteside and Sunter 2000). HIV attacks
two forms of the body's white blood cells, or CD4 cells, the T-cells and
macrophages, both of which are crucial for maintaining a functioning
immune system (Whiteside and Sunter 2000). AIDS occurs when, after
a number of years, T-cells and macrophages have declined to the extent
that the body is no longer capable of fighting off infection. A person is
generally said to have AIDS either when their CD4 count[4] drops below
200 or they begin to display signs of opportunistic infections or Kaposi's
sarcoma.

The fact that AIDS, rather than being a specific disease, is comprised
of a raft of associated diseases has made defining and diagnosing the
syndrome problematic. The American Food and Drug Administration (FDA) approved the first HIV-antibody test in 1985. However, testing remained a slow, expensive and complex process for much of the
1980s and 1990s. It was only as of 2002 that a rapid blood test, capable
of producing a result in 20 minutes, was devised. Further advances
have seen the FDA authorize a 'home testing kit', which is available
to Americans *via* the internet or local pharmacies (Waxman 2008).
However, testing in less developed countries, particularly in the early
days of HIV/AIDS, provided significant challenges in terms of both cost
and logistics. The absence of antibody tests necessitated alternative
means of diagnosis. In 1985, following a workshop in Bangui in the
Central African Republic, the World Health Organization (WHO 1986)
attempted a clinical case definition of AIDS. This definition was to
form the basis for diagnosis in poorer countries that did not possess a
developed diagnostic capacity. It is worth quoting at length in order
demonstrate the difficulties posed:

> AIDS in an adult is defined by the existence of at least two of the
> major signs associated with at least one minor sign, in the absence

of known causes of immunosuppression such as cancer or severe malnutrition or other recognised etiologies:

(1) *Major Signs* (a) weight loss >10% of body weight (b) chronic diarrhoea >1 month (c) prolonged fever >1 month (intermittent or constant).

(2) *Minor Signs* (a) persistent cough for >1 month (b) generalised pruritic dermatitis (c) recurrent herpes zoster (d) oro-pharyngeal candidiasis (e) chronic progressive and disseminated herpes simplex infection (f) generalised lymphadenopathy.

The presence of generalised Kaposi's sarcoma or cryptococcal meningitis are sufficient by themselves for the diagnosis of AIDS.

Further refinements were made in 1986, 1987, 1989, 1993, 1994, 1997, and 2000 (WHO 2009d). These adjustments illustrate the difficulties faced by healthcare professionals as they sought to come to terms with the illusive nature of AIDS.

Detecting evidence of HIV in the body has proved similarly problematic. Before notable advances in testing took place after 2000, Whiteside and Sunter (2000) described the process as looking for 'footprints on a sandy beach'. The aim was to locate evidence of an individual's past HIV infection, rather than find proof of the virus itself. Even in 2010, standard HIV tests were operating through the identification of HIV antibodies, rather than through evidence of the virus itself. These difficulties, alongside the necessarily arbitrary way in which AIDS is defined, have provided ammunition for those who query the existence of HIV/AIDS as a new condition, arguing that it is simply a 'new name for old diseases' (Whiteside and Sunter 2000).

'Plague' and the language of HIV/AIDS

In sub-Saharan Africa, HIV/AIDS is more than a disease. It is a complex social and political issue, and responses to it have necessarily incorporated biomedical, moral, cultural and governance elements in a way that other mass killers like malaria and tuberculosis, which annually claim one million and half a million African victims respectively, have not (WHO 2006b). As outlined, malaria has been responsible historically for far more fatalities than HIV/AIDS and yet receives a fraction of the attention. The 'language of AIDS' can be instructive in this regard. The 'Black Death' that swept through Europe during the latter part of the fourteenth century has been proffered frequently as a historical precedent to HIV/AIDS (Marks 2002). Former US President Bill Clinton

(2001) argued in a lecture organized by the National AIDS Trust that the 'world is facing its biggest plague since ... Europe lost a quarter of its people in the 14th century'. The United Nations (2004) has made similar pronouncements:

> Since 1981, when the first cases of AIDS were diagnosed, AIDS-related mortality has reached orders of magnitude comparable to those associated with visitations of pestilence in earlier centuries. The Black Death of 1347–1351 killed more than 20 million people in Europe; by the end of 2002, 22 million people had lost their lives to AIDS.

Similarly, it has been argued in the *British Medical Journal* that 'in terms of morbidity and mortality, the HIV/AIDS pandemic is worse than the Black Death of the 14th century' (Makgoba *et al* 2002). Alwyn Young (2004), currently of the London School of Economics, has created a model of the effects of the HIV/AIDS pandemic on South Africa based on a medieval plague scenario, arguing that 'in considering the economic consequences of the AIDS epidemic, one is drawn to historical examples of similar demographic catastrophes, perhaps the most well researched of which is the Black Death in Britain in the late 14th century'. In 'The Gift of the Dying: The Tragedy of AIDS and the Welfare of Future African Generations', he argues that the economic consequences of HIV/AIDS, like the Black Death, might be beneficial for those who survive.

The mortality rate associated with the Black Death was as high as 90 percent. Victims experienced grapefruit-sized boils, or buboes (hence 'bubonic' plague), loss of breath and continuous vomiting (Allen 2000). In Italy, Florence experienced eight episodes of the plague between 1340 and 1427, reducing the great city to a quarter of its pre-plague population. The average life expectancy during this period was halved, falling to below 20 years (Allen 2000). Some estimates (Frank 1999) suggest that England and Wales lost nearly 50 percent of their pre-plague populations in an 18-month period between 1348 and 1350. However, the extent to which the Black Death and HIV/AIDS merit comparison is debatable both in terms of geography and epidemiology. The most obvious distinction is the speed at which death occurs; the Black Death killed with incredible swiftness, unlike AIDS which, thanks to medicinal advances, can take decades. A far better comparison is syphilis; it kills slowly, it is sexually transmitted, it disproportionately affects the sexually-active 15–44 demographic and can be passed on *via* mother-to-child transmission (Chapter 1). However, where HIV/AIDS is concerned, the concept of 'the plague' has endured, and with it, a sense of impending doom that has not been associated with, for instance, malaria.

A 'gay plague'

From the outset, ignorance, fear and a general lack of understanding of the nature of HIV/AIDS and its transmission have proved part-and-parcel of the disease, exacerbating the difficulties experienced by sufferers and those around them. AIDS itself first came to the attention of the public in the US in 1981: unusually high clusters of occurrences of pneumocystis pneumonia, which causes lung infections in people with compromised immune systems, and Kaposi's sarcoma, a cancer caused by the human herpesvirus 8, were discovered in New York and California. All of the sufferers were young homosexual men. Before the disease was categorized by the Centre for Disease Control and Prevention as AIDS, it had begun to be referred to as the 'gay plague', 'gay pneumonia' or, more officiously, 'Gay Related Immune Deficiency' (Samuel and Engel 1988). The isolation of HIV as the virus responsible for AIDS came in 1984, three years after the 'discovery' of AIDS. Credit for the discovery of HIV was, after much academic jostling, eventually shared by Robert Gallo of the (US) National Institute of Health and Luc Montagnier of the (French) Pasteur Institute. In 2008, interest in this long-dormant tale of medical rivalry was rekindled when Montagnier and his colleague from the Pasteur Institute, Françoise Barré-Sinoussi, were awarded the Nobel Prize in Physiology or Medicine for their work on isolating HIV. Controversially, Gallo's role was passed over (*Science* 10/10/2008, *Scientific American* 06/10/2008).

In the early days of the HIV/AIDS epidemic, when most of the world's attention was focused on its impact in developed countries, homosexual men increasingly became a 'special area of study' for medical practitioners. An article in the *British Medical Bulletin* in 1988 analyses HIV/AIDS-related changes in perceptions of sex and sexuality:

> The conceptualisation of AIDS in terms of the groups most affected by it has largely determined the impact of the epidemic. Even medical science has been affected, as AIDS has forced many in the medical profession to come to terms with certain aspects of male homosexual mores and behaviour that were previously ignored. There can be few medical schools where AIDS has not meant a much greater awareness of homosexuality, indeed of sexuality in general ... It is difficult to speak of the impact of AIDS without speaking of the changing

perceptions of homosexuality and homosexuals, so intertwined are the two in the public imagination. AIDS seems to have increased simultaneously both the stigma and the respectability of homosexuals and in unravelling what may seem a contradiction we can come to terms with certain crucial social changes (Altman 1988).

Due to its association with the gay community, public sympathy for AIDS victims in the US tended to be low. A national survey conducted by the *Journal of the American Medical Association* in 1988 reflects the homophobic attitudes of the time. Of the respondents, 60 percent claimed 'not much' or 'no' sympathy for those who contracted HIV through homosexual intercourse. Twenty percent of those questioned maintained that sufferers 'were getting their rightful due' (study cited in Allen 2000). Similarly, a study published in the *American Journal of Public Health* showed that as late as 1991, up to a third of Americans surveyed claimed to be in favour of quarantining those with HIV/AIDS (Herek *et al* 2002). By 1999, almost 20 years after the discovery of AIDS, nearly 17 percent of respondents exhibited feelings of 'anger or disgust' towards people living with HIV (Herek *et al* 2002). The response of politicians and policymakers mirrored that of the public. In a seminal, emotionally-charged early history of HIV/AIDS in America, *And the Band Played On*, Randy Shilts (1987) raged against the slow response of the Reagan administration (1981–1989), the scientific community and the media to the growing epidemic confronting the gay community. He argued that the 'bitter truth was that AIDS did not just happen to America – it was allowed to happen'. As Shilts saw it, the spread of HIV/AIDS was facilitated by a government that refused to allocate sufficient funding to addressing the developing pandemic, by scientists who perceived there to be little kudos to be gained from studying a condition affecting homosexuals and by the popular media, which shied away from stories publicizing gay issues. However, Shilts reserved most of his ire for Reagan himself, describing him as 'the man who had let AIDS rage through America, the leader of the government that when challenged to action had placed politics above the health of the American people'. There is no doubt that Reagan largely ignored the disease until 1987, when he made his first public reference to HIV/AIDS in a speech establishing the Presidential Commission on the Human Immunodeficiency Virus (HIV) Epidemic. Even then, Reagan's speech touched on the dangers posed to haemophiliacs, to the recipients of blood transfusions and to the sexual partners of intravenous drug users, but did not once refer to the gay community that had borne the brunt of the disease and campaigned so hard for a governmental response (Shilts 1987). In taking this approach, the Reagan administration set the tone for the wider political response to the disease: prevaricate and delay. In 1987, Reagan's Secretary of Education, William J Bennet, claimed that AIDS demonstrated how 'harsh nature becomes the unwitting ally of responsible morality' (cited in Allen 2000).

It was only when it became apparent that HIV/AIDS was far from solely a 'minority' disease that the American government (and public) began to take it more seriously. In 1984, a 13-year-old haemophiliac from Indiana, Ryan White, was diagnosed as HIV-positive. He had become infected through the use of contaminated blood products. His desire to continue to live a normal life put perceptions of HIV/AIDS under the spotlight. White, according to the perspectives of the time, was an 'innocent victim'. His case forced Americans to begin to confront the discriminatory nature of their original ideas and to revise the ways in which they had engaged previously with HIV/AIDS. At the behest of local authorities and parents, White was initially barred from attending school. Even after he had secured readmission following an arduous appeals process, parents of other children sued (ultimately unsuccessfully) to prevent his return (Gilman 1987). The Ryan White story generated a media storm and helped transform attitudes towards HIV/AIDS. Other high-profile cases that served to modify the US approach to HIV/AIDS include those of the three Ray brothers from Florida, who were diagnosed as HIV-positive in 1986. Like Ryan White, they were haemophiliacs who had contracted the virus as a result of blood transfusions. A court victory allowing them readmission to their local school had resulted in the family home being firebombed (Allen, J. 2005). The erstwhile 'gay plague' began to be constructed as an affliction that could affect anyone.

Locating the origins of HIV

Clearly, the origins of HIV/AIDS are important to scientists engaged with understanding and combating it. However, it is the political dimension of the debate that has shaped the responses of African elites concerned with the governance of HIV/AIDS. Conspiracy theories surrounding the origins of HIV/AIDS abound and these have had a profound influence on political responses in countries like South Africa (Chapter 4). Even mainstream debates about the geographical origins of HIV/AIDS have proved hugely emotive for political elites wishing to dilute the stereotypical outsider view of sub-Saharan Africa as a region defined by disease and death. Yet it is precisely the fact that HIV/AIDS had its origins in Africa that offers analysts one of the simplest explanations for the rapid evolution of the pandemic; Western Equatorial Africa represents the epicentre of the HIV/AIDS pandemic (Iliffe 2006). Furthermore, arguments regarding the extent to which HIV/AIDS developed as a colonial-era iatrogenic event resonate with arguments stressing the obduracy of the colonial legacy in the shaping of contemporary Africa.

An archived serum sample, one of 672 collected in 1959 by a malaria researcher in Leopoldville in the Democratic Republic of Congo (then the Belgian Congo), has produced the earliest evidence of HIV (Iliffe 2006). There have also been attempts at retrospective diagnoses of people suffering from Kaposi's sarcoma and pneumocystis pneumonia – symptoms so common in AIDS sufferers – in sub-Saharan Africa in the late 1950s and 1960s. However, no blood samples from these individuals have survived. Nonetheless, the HIV-positive sample from 1959, since it was one of nearly 700 collected in the Leopoldville area at that time, shows that HIV was present in the Congo by the late 1950s, although by no means common (Korber *et al* 2000; Yusim *et al* 2001). It is now almost universally accepted by scientists that HIV originated from SIV (Hahn *et al* 2000; Sharp *et al* 2000), yet why and how SIV mutated into a human virus by 1959 remains largely unexplained. At the same time, the fact that diseases jump from animals to humans is well known. Some of humankind's most common afflictions – including measles, smallpox, tuberculosis, typhus, Dengue fever, yellow fever and 'Spanish flu' – are derived from human interaction with animals, with the species jump frequently having occurred thousands of years ago (Weiss 2001b see Table 2.1).

It is possible that SIV pre-dates HIV/AIDS by millions of years (Marx *et al* 2001). Given, then, that in equatorial Africa humans, chimpanzees

Table 2.1   **Human Infectious Diseases of Animal Origin**

Disease	Animal Source	Date of 'Jump'
Measles	Sheep/goat	*Ca.*6000 BCE
Smallpox	Ruminant?	>2000 BCE
Tuberculosis	Ruminant?	>1000 BCE
Typhus	Rodent	430 BCE/1492 CE
Plague	Rodent	541 CE/1347 CE/1665 CE
Dengue	Monkey	*Ca.*1000 CE
Yellow Fever	Monkey	1641 CE
Spanish Flu	Bird, Pig	1918 CE

Source: (Weiss 2001b)

and other primates have interacted for millennia, HIV's twentieth-century origin appears decidedly atypical. What seems clear, however, is that west and central Africans transported to America as slaves were not infected by any variant of SIV. There is no historical evidence of mass clusters of the opportunistic infections and diseases associated with AIDS (Marx 2005; Moore 2004). This is problematic for proponents of the zoonosis or 'cut-hunter' theory, who argue that hunters butchering chimpanzees and sooty mangabeys became infected with SIV through cuts on their hands, after which the virus, harmless to humans for centuries, mutated into HIV (Moore 2004). However, cut-hunter transmissions must have taken place at many points throughout the millennia of human-primate interaction. There are contemporary precedents: a 1996 Ebola hemorrhagic fever outbreak in Gabon was precipitated by the butchering of chimpanzees; 21 of the 37 people who were involved in the butchering and consumption of the 'bushmeat' subsequently died of the fever (Weiss 2003). Likewise, there are many recorded incidents of simian diseases being passed on to laboratory workers and pet owners (Weiss 2001a). A number of these diseases have proved dangerous to humans: monkeypox and filovirus are two of the more well known examples (Osterhaus 2001). It is argued that SIV might conceivably have made the jump on a number of occasions over the centuries but that infections petered out due to low rates of transmission and the isolation of the populations concerned (Weiss 2001b). It is certainly probable that HIV would have remained confined to the forests of its origin had it not been for the growing twentieth-century trend towards urbanization. There are other problems, too, with respect to the simian origin of HIV. As a result of a continuing reliance on 'bushmeat' across large parts of the continent, people in sub-Saharan Africa continue to be exposed to a number of strains of SIV. If the cut-hunter hypothesis is correct, the possibility remains that novel outbreaks of HIV may yet occur (Van Heuverswyn and Peters 2007).

Human agency and the origins of the virus

While the cut-hunter theory remains the most accepted explanation for the jump from SIV to HIV, there is sufficient evidence to suggest that the role of human agency in the creation of the HIV/AIDS pandemic should at least be considered. Inevitably, this point has attracted conspiracy theorists. For example, it has been argued that HIV/AIDS was created and spread deliberately by either the CIA or the South African apartheid regime, possibly with the intention of decimating African populations and enabling the West to appropriate Africa's wealth (Rödlach 2006). However, even without engaging with either this or any other conspiracy theory, it remains possible to make a case for human agency (as is reflected in the decision, in 2001, by the Royal Society of London to stage a high-profile public debate on the origins of HIV).

Both Brian Martin (2001) and Julian Cribb (2001) have asked why, in the absence of any hard evidence, the cut-hunter hypothesis has been so rapidly accepted as orthodoxy. Contentiously, they have argued that the evolution of SIV into HIV could not have been simply an 'act of God'. While their views are by no means generally accepted, their arguments speak to those wishing to find a 'rational' explanation for HIV/AIDS. A number of authors, including Louis Pascal (1991), Tom Curtis (1992), Walter Kyle (1992) and Edward Hooper (1999) have all linked the spread of HIV/AIDS to polio vaccination campaigns conducted in West Equatorial Africa during the later stages of the colonial period. All four authors have argued that the live polio vaccine administered to an estimated 900,000 people (Moore 2004) in the Belgian Congo (Democratic Republic of Congo) and Ruanda-Urundi (Rwanda and Burundi) in the late 1950s, was, having been cultivated in simian tissue, infected with SIV. While this has proved to be yet another of the controversial arguments surrounding the origins of HIV, simian diseases have indeed been passed on to humans through vaccinations in the past – the most notorious example of this being SV40, a simian virus that can cause brain tumours and cancer in humans (Cribb 2001; Weiss 2001a). The early proponents of the colonial vaccine theory, including Pascal (1991), Curtis (1992) and Kyle (1992), have been discredited: the simian tissue used to create the polio vaccines did not come from chimpanzees, which remain the accepted source of SIV. However, in *The River*, Hooper (1999) argued that chimpanzee cells were indeed used in the propagation of the polio vaccine, pointing to a chimpanzee colony maintained by the polio mission in the Belgian Congo. At the same time, a number of new facts relating to Hooper's hypothesis have subsequently come to light. Firstly, a batch of extant samples from the relevant vaccine were tested and found to be free of both SIV and chimpanzee tissue (Moore 2004). Secondly, a study published by scientists operating out of the Los Alamos National Laboratory produced a 'look-back' estimate for HIV-1 to 1930. Allowing for an error of 20 years on either side, the estimate dates the origin of HIV at between 1910 and 1950. This period pre-dates the live polio vaccine programme (Burr *et al* 2001). Despite Hooper sticking to his guns (his website, AIDS-Origins.com, continues to promote the theory), his argument has been largely dismissed.

At the same time, some level of support for an iatrogenic origin (induced inadvertently by either medical treatment or procedures, or the activity of healthcare professionals) remains. Preston Marx *et al* (2001) suggest that the rapid transformation of ancient SIVs into HIV can only be explained adequately by virtue of a modern intervention. They argue that it is unlikely that a 'naturally' occurring infection of a human host with SIV could have been the cause of the species-jump, because the human body would quickly overcome the infection – hence other factors must have been involved. Marx *et al* (2001) argue that one plausible explanation may be the use of unsterilized needles in mass vaccination and medical programmes. Hypodermic syringes, prior to the invention of plastic disposable units, were expensive, costing as much in 1900 as $50 in modern terms (Marx *et al* 2001). In 1918, only 100,000 syringes worldwide were being produced each year, but technological advances meant that this output had, by 1952, increased to eight million units per year. This rapid rise was partly due to the discovery of penicillin, which began to be produced for the mass market during the 1940s. The period also saw the advent of the welfare state and the emergence of national health systems in countries like Britain. Sheer increase in demand led to calls for cheaper syringes and, eventually, to the manufacture of a 'single-use', disposable syringe. By 1960, nearly one billion syringes were being produced globally on an annual basis, at a cost of 18¢ per syringe (Marx *et al* 2001). As their name suggests, 'single-use' syringes were supposed to be used once and then disposed of; they were not designed to be sterilized. However, despite the rapidly falling price of syringes, efforts to keep costs down meant that disposable syringes were reused. This remained the case until relatively recently. Prior to 1998, WHO guidelines allowed for the reuse of a single syringe up to 200 times if certain sterilizing procedures took place. However, WHO surveys indicate that such procedures were frequently not adequately employed (Drucker *et al* 2001).

The scale of injections administered in Africa during the 1950s was unparalleled. UNICEF alone oversaw the administration of over 35 million inoculations for yaws in central Africa during the 1950s and early 1960s (Drucker *et al* 2001). Colonial authorities, seeking desperately to justify their continued presence on the continent, rolled out mass vaccination programmes (Schneider 2009). Given the linkage between the management of African disease and wider social control in the years immediately prior to decolonization, it is possible to be cynical about some of the political motivation behind these programmes. However, as treatment and prevention programmes many were remarkably successful. At the same time, it is also possible that collectively they provided the perfect iatrogenic event for the evolution of SIV into HIV. As stated, the human body would ordinarily be expected to fight off an SIV with some success; simian viruses are poorly adapted for survival in human hosts. Significantly, though, if the virus had been present in sections of a population then the use of unsterilized needles may have facilitated a 'serial-passaging' (Moore 2004). By exposing SIV to a far wider array of human hosts than could ever have occurred naturally, the virus may have been given the opportunity to mutate into HIV (Moore 2004).

The heterosexual transmission of HIV is, relatively speaking, rather inefficient, at a rate of between just 0.01 and 0.2 percent. Blood transfusion, however, has an efficiency of approximately 90 percent. Between 1940 and 1960, a significant number of 'blood banks' were established in colonial Africa. Given that HIV is known to have been present in Kinshasa by 1959, its spread could well have been facilitated greatly by the routine use of transfusions in medical procedures. The then Belgian Congo was one of the earliest colonies to acquire a transfusion service, initiating its first programme in 1923. By 1955, a total of 19 African colonies had established transfusion services (Schneider and Drucker 2006). In addition to blood loss, transfusions were used to treat severe anaemia and dehydration in children. The number of transfusions rose from approximately 68,000 per year across the region in the 1940s, to approximately one million per year in the 1970s and to over two million per year in the 1980s (Schneider and Drucker 2006). By the time screening for HIV became available in the mid-1980s, an estimated 30–40 million blood transfusions had taken place. In combination, the mass vaccination programmes and transfusion services introduced by the colonial powers arguably point to a 'non-Darwinian' model for the incubation and spread of HIV/AIDS, if not specifically for its origin.

Charting the African pandemic

It is possible to argue that because HIV/AIDS originated in Africa, it is only natural that the continent has borne the brunt of the virus. Yet, while this might be the case for central Africa, it certainly does not hold for regions like southern Africa, parts of which received at least some warning that a potential pandemic was at hand. For example, South Africa had a prevalence rate of less than 1 percent in 1990 compared to that of 30 percent in parts of Uganda and Rwanda (Caraël and Glynn 2007; Gilbert and Walker 2002). Evidence suggests that the initial spread of HIV/AIDS was relatively slow, especially within rural areas. For 1959, we have that one HIV-positive sample from the Belgian

Congo. Over a decade later, in 1970, stored samples from 805 pregnant women in Kinshasa indicate the existence of just two HIV-positive individuals within the group (Iliffe 2006). By the late 1970s, however, doctors in Kinshasa were beginning to notice a dramatic increase in the prevalence of both Kaposi's sarcoma and cases involving severe wasting and diarrhoea. By the early 1980s, HIV/AIDS, as yet unidentified and unnamed, was entrenched firmly within the general population around Kinshasa. In 1985, samples drawn from over 5,000 subjects in Kinshasa showed 5 percent of donors were HIV-positive (Schoepf 2002). A study amongst sex workers in the same year demonstrated an infection level of 27 percent. A wider survey two years later revealed a prevalence of 35 percent (Schoepf 2002). Outside Kinshasa, progression was slower. Of 659 stored blood samples extracted from people from one village in northern DRC in 1976, only five were HIV-positive: 0.8 percent of the total village population. Blood samples taken from the same village a year later demonstrated an unchanged degree of infection (Iliffe 2006).

Over the course of the 1980s, HIV spread steadily outwards from the epicentre of Kinshasa. It moved up- and downstream of the capital and appeared in Gabon, the Central African Republic and Cameroon from the early 1980s onwards. It spread eastwards to Rwanda, Burundi, Uganda and Tanzania. (It may even have been present in parts of Uganda in the late 1970s.) By 1988, nearly 30 percent of the adult population in Kigali was infected (Caraël 2006). By the late 1980s, prevalence amongst sex workers in certain areas of Rwanda approached 80 percent (Caraël 2006). For those in central and east Africa, then, HIV/AIDS was *in situ* before it was properly identified. A number of countries in the region – Uganda, Senegal and Zaire – attempted aggressive anti-AIDS campaigns early on. Even so, to a certain extent at least, where these countries were concerned 'the horse had already bolted' and governments were faced with the task of suppressing an already rampant pandemic.

The situation in southern Africa was somewhat different. Southern Africa was more latterly exposed to the growing pandemic, but once HIV took hold in the region, it did so with a vengeance. Evidence from two mass campaigns against leprosy and tuberculosis undertaken in Malawi in 1981–1984 and 1987–1989 highlight the relative speed at which the disease advanced southwards. As part of the campaigns, blood samples were taken from 44,150 villagers in the Karonga district in the north of Malawi. Subsequently tested for HIV, the samples offer a window into the progression of the pandemic. Out of the initial group of 12,979 specimens, only eleven were found to be HIV-positive (Glynn *et al* 2001). Of the later specimens from the period 1987–1989, 189 were infected, a rise from 0.1 to 2 percent (Glynn *et al* 2001). By 2002, prevalence in the region had reached 10–15 percent (McCormack *et al* 2002). By 2004, southern Africa was home to nearly a third of the world's HIV/AIDS population. Yet, in contrast to the countries of central and eastern Africa, while some countries to the south were aware that they lay in the path of an encroaching pandemic, they still chose to do nothing about it.

By the mid-1980s, southern African states were coming into contact with HIV/AIDS. Zambia in particular was experiencing a significant number of infections, especially in the Copperbelt area, where copper mining draws migrant labourers. By 1985, approximately 8 percent of pregnant women in Lusaka were infected (Iliffe 2006). Botswana, Namibia and Zimbabwe only recorded their first cases of AIDS in 1985 or 1986, but subsequently experienced high levels of prevalence (Kaiser Family Foundation 2005b, 2005c, 2005d). By 2007, prevalence rates in these three countries amongst adults aged 15–49 were 23.9 percent, 15.3 percent and 15.3 percent respectively (UNAIDS 2008b). The experience of Lesotho, South Africa and Swaziland was somewhat different. It is tempting to argue that here, south of the Limpopo River, the effects of the pandemic could perhaps have been mitigated. Both Lesotho and Swaziland recorded their first cases of AIDS in 1986. Two decades later, these countries were at the centre of the pandemic, with prevalence rates amongst adults aged 15–49 reaching 23.2 percent and 26.1 percent respectively (UNAIDS 2008b). Similarly, by 2007, South Africa was experiencing HIV prevalence rates of 18.1 percent (UNAIDS 2008b). While it is doubtful whether HIV/AIDS could have been fully averted, statistics suggest that a window of opportunity existed in which preparations for the coming onslaught might have been made, especially by the South African authorities.

The earliest cases of HIV in South Africa conformed more to the Western model of infection than that beginning to sweep through the rest of sub-Saharan Africa. Although the first case of AIDS in South Africa was reported as early as 1982, early cases mirrored the American and European experience. Victims tended to be white homosexual men and people of both sexes who had received blood transfusions (Gilbert and Walker 2002). By 1990, homosexual men, nearly all of them white, accounted for 207 out of the 308 reported AIDS cases in South Africa (Gilbert and Walker 2002; Iliffe 2006). Evidence from community surveys shows that in the mid-1980s in KwaZulu-Natal (the South African province with the highest rate of prevalence post-2000) there was little evidence of HIV within the general population (Gilbert and Walker 2002). Likewise, tests conducted in Johannesburg in 1985 involving 522 samples found no evidence of HIV. Tests conducted on South African mineworkers in 1986 showed a prevalence of just 0.02 percent (Iliffe 2006). HIV/AIDS only became a heterosexual disease in South Africa after 1990; it was only then that its infection statistics began to mirror those of other African countries. With an HIV prevalence of over 30 percent in KwaZulu-Natal by 2009, it is clear that from these slow beginnings the virus moved through the population rapidly. The central debate – the counterfactual at the heart of the South African HIV/AIDS crisis – is whether, had the government been more willing, HIV/AIDS could have been prevented from gaining a foothold in South Africa. Shula Marks (2002) argues that 'HIV/AIDS was a pandemic waiting to happen in South Africa'. With migrant labour being blamed for the explosion of syphilis in South Africa in the early part of the twentieth century (Chapter 1) this system, established to service the mines, had long been viewed as a threat to public health. In 1949, Sidney Kark (2003), the medical doctor and academic, commented that migrant labour constituted the single greatest threat to health in South Africa at the time. The fact that HIV/AIDS spread so rapidly throughout South Africa and neighbouring 'labour pools' such as Lesotho and Swaziland, is evidence of just how prescient Kark's conclusions were.

Conclusion

That HIV/AIDS originated in sub-Saharan Africa and that the region has suffered disproportionately from its effects is undeniable. While its origins are arguably less important than combating it, it is important to accept that Africa is 'ground zero' where the pandemic is concerned. However, while this is a relatively neat explanation for the ferocity with which the pandemic unleashed itself here, it is not sufficient. Firstly, given the possibility of an iatrogenic explanation for the origin of HIV/AIDS, human agency has potentially been central to this story, and continues to be so. Secondly, attitudes towards the disease and its containment have been shaped by a number of factors, including political direction from above. Nearly 30 years after the first cases of AIDS were diagnosed in Africa, misinformation, prejudice and ignorance remain rife. Given that HIV/AIDS is the leading cause of death in sub-Saharan Africa and, increasingly, the major focus of aid agencies and international donors, it is important to get to grips with its origins, its social pathology and its cultural context. Notions of 'plague' and sexual 'deviancy' as well as a tendency to identify scapegoats are all symptomatic of the HIV/AIDS narrative to date. This book is concerned with the politics and governance of HIV/AIDS in sub-Saharan Africa. For this reason, it pays particular attention to the ways in which structures and institutions may have contributed to the rampant spread of HIV/AIDS. It is also concerned with people's reactions to HIV/AIDS, at both a political and a grassroots level. Subsequent chapters will deal with the socio-political implications of the development of a continental AIDS crisis and the resulting reorientation of the African development agenda towards combating a single disease.

3
Gender, Violence and the Spread of HIV/AIDS

HIV/AIDS has spread across much of Africa with chilling speed. In this respect, gender inequality is the proverbial elephant in the room. As with so many issues calling complex cultural norms into question, the very linkage of HIV/AIDS with the realities of African gender relations is emotive and disquieting; analysis is fraught with difficulty on a number of levels. At the same time, it is a fact that heterosexual transmission is, epidemiologically, at the heart of the HIV/AIDS pandemic, and African women appear to be disproportionately vulnerable to infection. It is therefore critical to consider very seriously the association between gender inequality and HIV/AIDS. There is no doubt that gender-based violence and HIV/AIDS in much of sub-Saharan Africa can be said to be almost symbiotic; the two strands tend to be mutually reinforcing. However, while Kofi Annan, then Secretary-General of the United Nations, described AIDS in Africa as having 'a woman's face' (Annan 2002), debates about gender hierarchies, sexual and physical violence, cultural norms and human rights all sit rather uncomfortably beneath this particular rubric. Gender-based analysis of HIV/AIDS in sub-Saharan Africa, particularly studies conducted by 'outside' NGOs and agencies, has provoked a backlash from African leaders like Thabo Mbeki (2004), who equate perceived criticisms of African norms and values by bodies like the New York-based NGO Human Rights Watch (1995, 1997, 2001, 2002, 2003 and 2004) with cultural imperialism.

The inference that gender-based violence has accelerated the spread of HIV/AIDS has stirred considerable controversy. However, it is difficult to counter the argument that violence against women facilitates the spread of HIV/AIDS and that HIV/AIDS, likewise, contributes to increased levels of violence against women. Statistics from across the continent tell a grim tale. In conflict zones like the DRC, sexual assault used as a 'weapon of war' by combatants resulted in nearly 16,000 cases of rape in 2008; the majority of victims were adolescent girls (HRW 2009). Likewise, in Darfur, reports of mass rape indicate that sexual assault formed an integral aspect of the violence perpetrated by agents of the Sudanese state (HRW 2007, 2008). There is also evidence of institutionalized rape in previous, and in some cases ongoing, conflict sites like Burundi, Central African Republic, Liberia, Rwanda, Sierra Leone and Northern Uganda (Amnesty International 2005). However, figures from non-combat zones are arguably more problematic, given that they afford a deeper insight into gender relations. A United Nations (2003) Office on Drugs and Crime report on southern Africa issued in 2003 described 'crimes related to violence against women, especially but not only rape, constitute a disturbing phenomenon that appears to be endemic in the region'. The report cited marked increases in sexual violence in Botswana, Lesotho, Namibia and Zimbabwe. A study published in *The Lancet* in 2009 suggested that a third of Swazi girls between the ages of 13 and 24 have been sexually assaulted (Murray and Burnham 2009). Similarly, in Zambia, one in eight teenage girls surveyed in 2002 claimed to have been forced into sex over the course of the previous year (UNAIDS 2004). However, even these disturbing figures are dwarfed by the levels of sexual violence in South Africa.

South Africa makes for a revealing case study in gender-based violence, given the significant disparity between the rights afforded women by the South African Constitution, and South African women's actual experiences. The constitution that formed the basis of the 'new' post-apartheid South Africa was admired worldwide for its emphasis on liberal democratic values and its inclusion of an 'equality clause' that offered increased protection for women. In addition, the South African government moved to engage with issues like women's representation in parliament; women MPs now constitute 43 percent of the total (Inter-Parliamentary Union 2010). This gives South Africa the distinction of having the third highest number of women MPs, trumped only by Sweden and Rwanda. Likewise, the country has vocal gender-focused elements within civil society. Following the first democratic elections in 1994, South Africans, as citizens of the most economically-developed country south of the Sahara, looked to put the violence and inequality of the apartheid era behind them. Fifteen years on, these changes have done little to free women from either the threat or the reality of gender-based violence. One possible explanation for this disparity, alongside, of course, the ongoing legacy of the brutalizing socio-political infrastructure of apartheid, is that advances in legal equality and political representation are simply a veneer concealing a culture in which entrenched gender hierarchies remain socially acceptable.

Across Africa, the strident calls for greater legislative protection for women are redundant if this continues to have little to no effect on women's day-to-day lives – and the gulf between legal niceties and the reality of women's experiences is stark. South Africa has achieved notoriety as the 'rape capital of the world'. A survey undertaken by the South African Medical Research Council in 2009 suggests that 25 percent of South African men have committed some form of rape (Jewkes *et al* 2009a). Almost half of those who admitted rape claimed to have carried out more than one assault and nearly 8 percent confessed to having raped more than ten victims. These statistics reflect a grassroots gender/power imbalance that is at odds with the increased visibility of women within the historically male political arena. Critically, however, at the state level, gender-based violence and the spread of HIV/AIDS are frequently problematized separately; the former as a 'human rights issue' and the latter as a 'health issue'. The framing of gender-based violence as a rights issue potentially glosses over underlying social and cultural 'norms' that are arguably causal factors.

The interface between gender-based violence and HIV/AIDS

According to the 2007 'HIV/AIDS/STI Strategic Plan for South Africa', just over 5.5 million South Africans were living with HIV in that year, of which approximately 55 percent were female (Department of Health 2007). The South African Department of Health's 2008 seropositivity figures for pregnant women indicate prevalence rates of 29.3 percent at the national level (Department of Health 2009). This average belies a significant degree of variation across the country, with a high of 38.7 percent in the province of KwaZulu-Natal, and a comparative low of 16.1 percent in the Western Cape (Department of Health 2009). Here is just one example of the potential difficulties inherent in generalizing about gender and HIV/AIDS in sub-Saharan Africa, even at a national level. At the same time, these figures are reflective of a continental trend across sub-Saharan Africa where women account for almost 60 percent of HIV infections (UNAIDS 2008b). Outside of sub-Saharan Africa, the gender ratio is closer to 50:50. However, these numbers alone do not convey the full story. Young women in South Africa are far more likely to contract HIV than their male cohorts: 90 percent of new infections amongst the 15–24 demographic are female (UNAIDS 2008a). In 2005, in the 20–29 demographic, HIV incidence was more than 600 percent higher amongst women than men of the same age. High incidence of HIV amongst men only becomes evident when they begin to approach their thirties (UNAIDS 2008a).

It is also young women and girls who tend to suffer most from sexual violence. Where violence against women is concerned, many of the statistics emanating from South Africa are disquieting. However, they bear repeating, if only to emphasize the sheer scale of the problem of men's power over women and children. As mentioned above, a 2009 survey by the South African Medical Research Council indicated that one in four South African men had perpetrated a rape (Jewkes *et al* 2009a). Likewise, evidence suggests that one third of South African women will be raped at some point in their lives, while a quarter will suffer violent domestic abuse (Moffett 2006). In 2004/05, the South African Police Service (SAPS 2005) recorded over 50,000 reported cases of rape. However, the SAPS has estimated that just 3 percent of actual rapes are ever reported. Even allowing for lower estimates of between 5 and 10 percent, it is possible, on these figures, to make an argument for approximately half a million cases of rape annually. In 2008/09, the SAPS (2009) recorded 71,500 cases of 'sexual offences' including rape, an increase of 12 percent over that of the previous year. Many of these assaults are on children (both male and female). Of the nearly 16,000 reported cases of child rape in 2001, nearly 40 percent of the victims were under the age of 11 (van Niekerk 2003). The notorious 'Baby Tshepang' case, which saw a 23-year-old man sentenced to life imprisonment for the rape of a nine-month-old baby, highlighted growing awareness of such assaults. SAPS statistics demonstrate that 52 percent of reported cases of indecent assault between 2007 and 2008 involved children (RAPCAN 2008). Under-reporting means that it is conceivable that, each year, up to 500,000 children are sexually abused in South Africa (RAPCAN 2008).

There is a strong correlation between intimate partner violence (IPV) and the spread of HIV/AIDS (Dunkle *et al* 2006). Evidence from countries including Rwanda, Tanzania and South Africa indicates that HIV-positive women are more likely to have suffered from IPV than women who were not infected. Given that IPV in South Africa appears to be commonplace, with over 30 percent of male respondents (aged 15–26) to a study in the Eastern Cape Province admitting to such behaviour, the ramifications become clear (Dunkle *et al* 2006). A report in the journal *AIDS* suggests that domestic violence, both sexual and physical, should be viewed as an 'independent risk factor' when determining the spread of HIV/AIDS amongst women. The two aspects are arguably linked because violent men have a propensity to engage in risky behaviours and are therefore more likely to become HIV-positive (Dunkle *et al* 2006). This hypothesis appears to be borne out by studies that show that, in comparison to men who do not rape, men who rape tend to have a higher number of sexual partners, and tend to begin having sex at a relatively young age. The study emphasizes how understanding cultural constructs of masculinity is central to combating both IPV and the spread of HIV/AIDS:

> culturally tailored interventions addressing intersections of violence perpetration and high-risk sexual behaviour among young men in South Africa are urgently needed, and we propose that these interventions must specifically target not just individuals but engage communities in transformative dialogue around ideals of masculinity (Dunkle *et al* 2006).

Some relationships, not necessarily physically violent, are based on entrenched gender hierarchies and are therefore also problematic where HIV/AIDS is concerned. 'Cross-generational' relationships, for example, whereby adolescent girls are involved in 'transactional' sexual relationships with significantly older men, are common across much of sub-Saharan Africa (Luke and Kurz 2002). In many instances the 'sugar daddies' are twice the girls' age (Silberschmidt and Rasch 2001). The girls involved in these relationships tend to have little bargaining power and are expected to 'pay' for their benefactors' largess. While such relationships may be consensual, vast disparities in wealth and status mean that the girls concerned have little 'power to negotiate safe sexual behaviours' (Luke and Kurz 2002). Furthermore, older men are far more likely to be infected with HIV than their adolescent male counterparts. An age difference of just five years significantly increases an adolescent girl's chances of contracting HIV (Hope 2007).

The extent to which the cultural construction of masculinities lies at the heart of the HIV/AIDS and gender debate is contentious in the extreme – and yet difficult to ignore. Female respondents in South Africa's Eastern Cape Province have described both gender-based violence and the spread of HIV/AIDS as 'all the fault of men' (Flint 2009i). Jewkes *et al* (2003) argue that 'for women social norms defining their acceptable behaviour, characteristics and responsibilities, economic dependency, and violence make them vulnerable, whereas ideals of masculinity associated with risk taking and sexual conquest also create vulnerability in men'. If gender-based violence, together with its causal links to the spread of HIV/AIDS, is embedded in socio-cultural norms, then any attempt to address the issue should focus on transforming the ways in which perceptions of gender are constructed. Instead, attempts by the South African government to prevent such violence have tended to be anchored in a rights-based discourse that bears little relevance to the realities of what it is to be a woman in South Africa.

Problematizing gender-based violence

The problem of gender-based violence is international. It is prevalent in rich and poor countries alike. The South African rights-based framework addressed above can be seen as an extension of attempts by the international community to problematize gender discrimination. From the 1970s, a number of international conferences were held, usually under the auspices of the United Nations, with the aim of formulating a rights-based response to gender discrimination. In 1979, the Convention on the Elimination of all forms of Discrimination against Women (CEDAW) marked an important milestone, successfully placing gender on the international agenda. However, somewhat paradoxically, the initial text of CEDAW did not address the issue of gender-based violence. This element of the convention was only introduced 13 years later, in 1992, in the shape of Resolution 19 (UN 1992). Resolution 19's influence was made evident a year later in 1993, when the UN World Conference on Human Rights produced the Vienna Declaration and Programme of Action, which was adopted by 171 states. The Vienna Declaration emphasized that 'the human rights of women and of the girl-child are an inalienable, integral and indivisible part of universal human rights' (UN 1993a). In so doing, the declaration defined violence against women as a violation of human rights. The UN (1993b) General Assembly reinforced this view in its Declaration on the Elimination of Violence against Women, which affirmed that 'violence against women constitutes a violation of the rights and fundamental freedoms of women and impairs or nullifies their enjoyment of those rights and freedoms'. In 1995, the Fourth World Conference on Women, held in Beijing, reiterated the idea of gender-based violence as a rights issue, declaring that 'violence against women both violates and impairs or nullifies the enjoyment by women of their human rights and fundamental freedoms' (UN 1995).

These conventions and declarations afforded gender issues a high international profile. However, there are a number of potential problems inherent in a 'human rights' approach to combating gender violence. Claims of universality notwithstanding, human rights have been criticized for articulating a Western view of the world (Ojo 1990). In the mid-1990s, feminists like Hilary Charlesworth (1995) began to argue that, as a concept, 'human rights' is a construct of a largely male perspective and that more is needed to be done to 'broaden the traditionally androcentric scope of rights'. The framework has also been criticized as neo-imperialist; an attempt by the North to assert its values over the South (Harris-Short 2003).

Questions, too, have been raised as to the efficacy of the legalistic approach inherent in the human rights framework, emphasizing as it does law and accountability when addressing the issue of violence against women. Jindy Jan Pettman (1996) has described human rights law as inherently 'gendered'. The use of gender-neutral language and an emphasis on gender equality – see the texts relevant to CEDAW, DEVAW and the Vienna Declaration – precludes acceptance of the special nature of the problem of violence against women (Kaufman and Lindquist 1995). According to this perspective, women face specific challenges that simply cannot be addressed by a legalistic framework centred on notions of 'equality'. Joan Fitzpatrick (1994), for example, makes the point that, for many women in abusive relationships, the problem is one of a dependency on violent men; equality before the law is not necessarily a remedy.

While gender-based violence is potentially universal in scope, it can take many forms. It is multifaceted, incorporating issues of class, race and religion. Reductionism can therefore be both difficult and dangerous (Mohanty 1991). Moreover, when it comes to discourse centred on 'Third World women', 'culture' is frequently the key focal point. In practice, the issue of 'culture' represents a minefield, especially when pertaining to issues of gender and violence, given the necessarily emotive nature of any debate surrounding charges of 'cultural essentialism' and 'the reification of culture' (Kapur 2002). Frequently-debated symbols of gender hierarchy across the world include the wearing of the veil, female genital cutting, dowry, lobola (bride price) and sati (the self-immolation of widows) (Krishnadas 2006). Debates on gender and HIV/AIDS are no less emotively fraught. Thabo Mbeki (2004) famously railed against the view that a misogynistic African culture somehow lies at the heart of the pandemic:

> I, for my part, will not keep quiet while others whose minds have been corrupted by the disease of racism accuse us as being ... by virtue of our Africanness and skin colour – lazy, liars, diseased, corrupt, violent, amoral, sexually depraved ... rapists.

Ratna Kapur's (2002) work on the 'victim subject' highlights how the discourse on gender-based violence has evolved to facilitate a focus on 'cultural explanations' – particularly 'intimate' story-telling by victims of domestic violence and sexual assault. The work of anti-prostitution groups, such as the Coalition against Trafficking in Women (CATW) that campaigns against the sex trade in developing countries, can from this perspective be seen to exacerbate the portrayal of women in the South as perpetual victims. Jo Doezema (2001) maintains that groups like CATW are responsible for the image of 'the kidnapped, raped, beaten, ill "third world prostitute" [who] stands as a powerful symbol for the exclusion of women from "universal" human rights due to their sexual subordination': the female body is constructed as a site of harm, and women as helpless victims; damaged 'others' in need of protection. The outcome of such discourse, even within feminist works, has arguably been the evolution of a paternalistic and somewhat condescending view of the 'Third World Woman':

> This average third world woman leads an essentially truncated life based on her feminine gender (read: sexually constrained) and being 'third world' (read: ignorant, poor, uneducated, tradition-bound, dom- estic, family-oriented, victimized, etc.). This, I suggest, is in contrast to the (implicit) self-representation of Western women as educated, modern, as having control over their own bodies and sexualities, and the freedom to make their own decisions (Mohanty 1991).

By assigning responsibility for the protection of women's bodies over to the state, human rights discourse arguably reinforces a paternalistic perspective towards women. This is also problematic in that an emphasis on state mechanisms does little to effect change in either power relations or gender hierarchies. Added to what is often a lack of effective capacity on the part of the state, this means that most 'human rights standards remain only words on a page, never being effectively implemented' (Fried 2003). The South African government has, through the auspices of the UN and the Southern African Development Community (SADC) res- pectively, ratified many international and regional resolutions on gender- based violence. For example 'The Prevention and Eradication of Violence against Women and Children' was signed by SADC heads of state in 1998. The South African Constitution, too, places a great deal of stress on the equality of women before the law, together with the right of the indi- vidual to control access to his/her person (Section 9 and Section 12). Nevertheless, as the above statistics suggest, such clauses have done little to protect South African women from either sexual assault or domestic violence. In essence, the 'legal formalization of rights and the establishment of legal machinery for their implementation makes the achievement of these forms an end in itself' (Kennedy 2002). This is not to argue that the state should not legislate to prevent gender-based violence, but rather that legalistic solutions are, on their own, wholly insufficient.

Human rights legislation in South Africa is, due to the inequities of apartheid, a relatively recent phenomenon. This, together with the vicious nature of the apartheid regime, means that it is relatively easy to make the claim that decades of brutalization, combined with a lack of experience with liberal conventions, has meant that the 'seeds' of the new rights agenda have fallen on stony ground. In addition, in many instances freedom from the oppression of apartheid prompted a desire to reassert 'traditional' African community values, which often ran counter to the liberal ideal enshrined in international human rights law. The result is that, despite the overwhelmingly liberal nature of the South African Constitution and its primacy over 'customary law', the rights enshrined therein have often had little impact on what David Kennedy (2002) has described as the 'background norms' determining sexual relations and gender hierarchies in South Africa. Kennedy (2002) argues further that '[h]uman rights remedies, even when successful, treat the symptoms rather than the illness, and this allows the illness not only to fester, but to seem like health itself. This is most likely where signing up for a norm against discrimination comes to substitute for ending the practice'. The reality is that the South African Constitution brings the promise of liberal and universal values, whilst precluding the emergence of alternative discourses that could potentially offer fresh insight into how best to engender real social change.

Politicizing HIV/AIDS and gender

In 1994, South Africans celebrated their country's first democratic election, which, it was understood, was ushering in a new society modelled on a rights-based framework. The ideal of complete equality and freedom for all citizens was enshrined in its new Constitution, which promised a transformation of society. Placing a significant degree of emphasis on equality, including gender equality, the Constitution committed the state to preventing abuse and to punishing abusers. One of the last acts of the apartheid regime was the passing of the Prevention of Family Violence Act which, for the first time, made marital rape a crime. This legislation formed the basis for the 1998 Domestic Violence Act, which described domestic violence as a 'serious social evil' and accepted that 'the remedies currently available to the victims of domestic violence have proved to be ineffective' (South African Government 1998). In 1996, the government established the Commission on Gender Equality (CGE), with the aim of ensuring that women were treated equally before the law (South African Government 1996b). However, as the post-apartheid era unfolded, it increasingly seemed that formal rights for women were established as an end in themselves, rather than as the foundation for a wider programme promoting equality. This had the effect of pigeonholing violence against women, placing it within a human rights context and effectively depoliticizing the issue. In contrast, HIV/AIDS rapidly became a political issue, especially once Thabo Mbeki became President of South Africa in 1999.

The political storm that followed Mbeki's AIDS scepticism (Chapter 4) resulted in the government debating the safety of AZT and seeking home-grown cures for AIDS. At the same time, rape survivors were being denied access to post-exposure prophylaxis (PEP).[1] In addition to filibustering about AIDS, the state's attitude towards the provision of PEP in the early days of Mbeki's presidency is illustrative of an unwillingness to address seriously violence against women. In this respect, a consequence (arguably unintentional) of the politicization of HIV/AIDS was that there was little simultaneous attempt to politicize rape, either as a conduit for HIV or as an issue in its own right. In 2002, the government eventually bowed to pressure to provide PEP for victims of sexual assault, although cynics argued that the timing of the PEP authorization, announced in the run-up to the 2004 general election, made it something of a public relations exercise.

The furore surrounding PEP obscured the pressing question of how levels of sexual violence had been allowed to spiral so out of control. Part of the problem is that continuously high levels of sexual violence have been deeply embarrassing for the government (Andrews 2007). Mbeki was vociferous in his criticism of those who placed South Africa's rape statistics under the spotlight. Targets of his ire included rape survivor, activist and freelance journalist Charlene Smith, and Deputy Executive Director of UNAIDS, Kathleen Cravero, both of whom he accused of racism and of portraying African men as 'violent sexual predators' (Mbeki 2004). Questions raised about the government's failure to control violent crime, including rape, were proof, in Mbeki's view, of a psychosis manifest in a number of white South Africans due to the 'psychological residue of apartheid' (Mbeki 2004). Any attempt to portray rape as in any way endemic was derided by Mbeki (2004) as an assault on African tradition and culture and an implication that 'African traditions, indigenous religions and culture prescribe and institutionalise rape'.

This can arguably be viewed as evidence once again of the South African state's commitment to a form of gender equality that is largely symbolic. This is because 'no human rights culture can effectively be established through legislative measures alone' (Greyling 2009). In 1996 the UN Special Rapporteur on Violence Against Women, Radhika Coomaraswamy (1997), argued that there was an urgent need for a 'complete overhauling of the criminal justice apparatus' to address the violence in South Africa, and 'violence against women in particular'. The 1998 Domestic Violence Act, while seemingly comprehensive on paper, was slow to be implemented, and little clarity was evident where budgets and training were concerned (Onyejekwe 2004). From the outset, there was a marked lack of political will to enforce the legislation; in 1999, Mbeki described South African rape statistics as 'purely speculative' (cited in Human Rights Watch 2001).

The conviction rates for rape demonstrate the minimal impact of women's human rights legislation on the South African courts: the rate of conviction with a custodial sentence is low compared to other violent crimes like murder, where successful prosecutions are far more plentiful (Leggett 2003). With reported rapes representing only a fraction of actual cases, conviction levels for rape are negligible. This, arguably, sends out a message that rape is not a 'serious' crime and that the risk of adverse consequences for rapists are relatively minor. The reaction to the 2006 trial of Jacob Zuma, who became President of South Africa in 2009, for allegedly raping an HIV-positive family friend, exposed some of the fault lines in the fight for gender equality in South Africa.[2] During the trial, massed Zuma supporters outside the court chanted 'burn the bitch' (Robins 2008), while ANC Youth leader Julius Malema, in response to questions about the case, declared that, because the complainant had not run away after the supposed act, she had clearly enjoyed the experience (Keehn 2009). Criticisms of Malema's remarks led to a charge against him being laid before the Equality Court which was established in 2005 to hear cases of discrimination. Malema described the court as 'Mickey Mouse' and dismissed the charge against him as being part of an attempt by white South Africans to 'embarrass the leadership' of the ANC. 'Progressive' forces, he said, should mobilize to expose this reactionary agenda.

President Zuma's polygamous marriages have led critics to fear that the political elite of the country is being seen to condone multiple concurrent partners (Flint 2009a, 2009b, 2009i). Debates surrounding the effects of polygamy on male 'promiscuity' in southern Africa have been numerous (see for example Andrews 2009; Delius and Glaser 2004; Spiegel 1991). Detractors argue that the practice has created an expectation that multiple sexual partners for men, formal and informal, is the norm. Zuma's public position on 'traditional' gender values has been frequently at odds with the spirit of the Constitution. In 2004, speaking in favour of 'virginity testing', in which girls are inspected by village matriarchs, Zuma described his wish for a return to the days when 'girls knew that their virginity was their family's treasure' (BBC 2004). His reference to Zulu 'tradition' in his rape defence also raised concerns amongst women's groups. He argued that the sex between him and his alleged victim was consensual and that 'in Zulu culture you cannot leave a woman if she is ready. To deny her sex, that would have been tantamount to rape' (Vincent 2009). That being said, over the course of his trial, it was clear that a significant percentage of Zuma supporters were women (Andrews 2009). Furthermore, despite the evidence presented at his trial, Zuma retained the support of the influential ANC Women's League, which went on to back him in his subsequent leadership struggle against Thabo Mbeki (Hassim 2009).

Jacob Zuma epitomizes the tensions between customary law and common law in South Africa. While the Constitution technically supersedes all forms of traditional law, it also accommodates 'other rights and freedoms that are recognized and conferred by common law, customary law or legislation, to the extent that they are consistent with the Bill' (South African Constitution, Chapter 2, Section 39). In reality, it is difficult to ensure consistency with the Bill as it is often customary systems, rather than legal niceties, that affect the way in which people are raised and the manner in which masculinities are fashioned. For instance, while gender equality is enshrined in the Constitution, Sotho customary law allows for husbands to beat their wives in order to discipline them (Pickup 2001). Andrews (2009) argues that 'feminist and human rights scholars and advocates have been reluctant to portray indigenous laws and institutions as antithetical to women's rights, appreciating that the characterization of such a binary often downplays the significance of a rights culture that is located within indigenous laws and institutions'. Nonetheless, that the framing of 'traditional' masculinity has become distorted is arguably exemplified by the rising number of 'corrective rapes' carried out against lesbians in South Africa (ActionAid 2009). While the full extent of this practice is difficult to quantify, a number of studies have made reference to what gender activists see as a worrying new trend (see for example ActionAid 2009; Harris 2004; Nel and Judge 2008).

While gender-based violence in South Africa is framed by the state in terms of human rights, the HIV/AIDS epidemic tends to be framed in terms of health, social welfare and, as former President Mbeki frequently emphasized, in terms of extreme poverty. Conceived of in this manner, the two streams rarely overlap, despite evidence of mutual reinforcement (Vetten and Bhana 2001). Where the two are viewed in conjunction by the state, gender-based violence tends to be categorized as merely a factor within the broader HIV/AIDS discourse rather than as a problem in its own right. Consequently, the South African state has been largely ineffectual in its dealings with both issues.

Gender-based violence and HIV/AIDS need to be framed as coexistent and mutually dependent variables of the same issue – gender inequality. In many instances, the links are self-evident. In any country with a significant HIV/AIDS population, coercive sex is likely to be a conduit for the spread of the disease, especially given that condoms tend not to be used in such encounters. In South Africa, that gang rape is a common form of sexual assault, accounting for 17.4 percent of assaults in a study of sexual violence in Gauteng Province, heightens the possibility of infection for the victim (Vetten *et al* 2008). Other studies from Johannesburg suggest that gang rape could constitute as much as 27 percent of all sexual assaults (Vetten and Haffejee 2005). Likewise, the sexual assault of minors, due to physiological reasons, carries a high likelihood of viral transmission; data suggest that approximately 40 percent of reported rapes are of youths under the age of 18 (Jewkes *et al* 2009b; South African Government 2007). The fear of violence is a further contributing factor. As victims within abusive relationships, many women feel unable to dictate condom use or withhold sex (Peacock and Levack 2004). There is also the increased risk of violence for women who have found themselves to be HIV-positive and have disclosed this information to partners and the community at large (Flint 2009a, 2009b, 2009c, 2009d, 2009e and 2009i).

Teenagers in South Africa's Eastern Cape Province indicate that sex is considered to be an area of male control and male power (Flint 2009f, 2009g, 2009h). Furthermore, the report by the South African Medical Research Council that highlighted that, conceivably, one in four South African men had committed rape, implies that fear of sanction has had little effect on curbing such instances of violent crime. With respect to the transmission of HIV/AIDS, evidence suggests that there is a correlation between violent and aggressive male behaviour in the home and the risk of HIV infection for women (Dunkle *et al* 2004). This is problematic, because intimate partner violence goes largely unremarked upon in many parts of South Africa. To an extent, violence is condoned, and excused, as 'inherently masculine' behaviour (Jewkes *et al* 2002).

Masculinity and the imposition of gender hierarchies

The legacy of colonialism, which reached its nadir in the apartheid regime that brutalized the population of South Africa for nearly 50 years, has been a frequently-proffered explanation for high levels of gender-based violence in Africa. Given that South Africa is, unlike the DRC, a non-conflict zone, it has a general 'culture of violence' that has been much commented upon in both the international and national media. The South African situation is the outcome of decades of institutionalized emasculation: 'Bantu education', dangerous working conditions, grown men being designated as 'boys' in the workplace and high levels of unemployment all served to drive male frustration, with only woman there to 'cushion against their complete powerlessness' (Ramphele cited in Marks and Andersson 1990). The system of migrant labour ensured the breakdown of traditional family life in many parts of the country, while debasing conditions on the mines and in the surrounding townships contributed to the development of a pervasive culture of violence (Marks 2002). It is therefore arguable that men have adopted an exaggerated form of masculinity – prioritizing risk-taking and violence – as a coping mechanism; a response to stress, uncertainty and danger (Outwater *et al* 2005). Much of this violence was, and remains, aimed at women. Research focused on rural areas of the Eastern Cape in the 1940s and 1950s reflects increased evidence of a longstanding 'war against women' (Mager cited in Marks 2002). As apartheid entered its last days in the late 1980s, levels of social disintegration burgeoned, with the removal of population control restrictions resulting in thousands moving to urban areas (Marks 2002). The collapse of the apartheid system saw an intensification of urbanization, with the resultant proliferation of impoverished 'informal urban areas'. This unravelling of the social fabric, together with the low-level war still being waged by the apartheid regime in the interests of suppressing dissent, ensured that violence, alienation and dislocation rapidly became hallmarks of South African life. The liberation movements also played their part in shaping South Africa's 'culture of violence'. In order to undermine apartheid, anti-apartheid organizations like the ANC were determined to make the townships 'ungovernable'. Perceived collaborators with the regime were punished publicly by their communities. Between January 1984 and August 1986, at the height of the state of emergency, nearly 350 people were 'necklaced'[3] by vigilante mobs in full view of the international press (Carstens 2003). Such strategies arguably sanctioned the view that violence offered an effective route to achieving political and social change.

Conclusion

The intersection of gender hierarchies, sexual violence and the spread of HIV/AIDS is apparent in sub-Saharan Africa. Efforts to combat the spread of HIV/AIDS will only begin to become effective once the social factors that make women susceptible to the disease are addressed. The fact that women, and predominantly younger women, in sub-Saharan Africa are so disproportionately affected by HIV/AIDS is symptomatic of a gendered climate of violence. HIV/AIDS and gender-based violence, when considered in isolation from each other, are frequently framed in very different ways. HIV/AIDS is viewed as a health issue and gender-based violence as a rights issue, meaning that the multiple points of connection between the two issues are frequently missed. Furthermore, the anchoring of debates concerning gender-based violence within a rights-orientated framework focuses attention on the individual perpetrators of crime rather than on the structures facilitating abuse. For any conceptualization of gender rights to be meaningful, the underlying causes of inequality and sexual violence must be addressed.

Internationally, there are increasing calls to legislate against gender-based violence. Where the exploration of the limits of rights-based discourses in guaranteeing equality and bodily integrity is concerned, South Africa is a critical arena. Here, the high levels of sexual violence and entrenched gender hierarchies juxtaposed against the strong legal and constitutional protection offered to women demonstrates how the adoption of international human rights discourse in terms of legislation and formal rights to address violence against women has largely failed. The South African government, whilst playing lip service to the idea of gender equality, has shown little evidence of political will to engage actively with the underlying problems that link the spread of HIV/AIDS with gender inequality and violence against women. Despite the state's role as a world leader with respect to women's representation in parliament, and its widely admired liberal constitution, its leadership has largely refused to deal with the complexities of problematic gender issues at a grassroots level. During his presidency, Thabo Mbeki argued that rape statistics were exaggerated and framed attempts to highlight cases of violence against women in terms of a racist agenda designed to denigrate African men. Likewise, the current president, Jacob Zuma, has made questionable statements regarding the 'traditional duties' of the Zulu man, and the transmission of HIV/AIDS, as has the leader of the African Youth League, Julius Malema, who dismissed the Equality Court as a 'Mickey Mouse' institution. Under conditions of gross gender inequality, continued references to equality under the law, human rights and the dignity of the individual are all largely meaningless. By addressing violence against women solely as a rights issue, the state has deflected uncomfortable questions pertaining to entrenched societal norms. The system as it stands is reactive rather than proactive, promising to punish perpetrators rather preventing violence in the first place. The advocation of behaviour change, safer sex, abstinence and fidelity (Chapters 6 and 7) are all very well when the individuals concerned have a choice in the dictation of their behaviour. However, high levels of sexual assault and physical violence against women and girls mean that the choices of many individuals are severely limited. The ramifications for the spread of HIV/AIDS have been significant.

4
Policymaking, Dissidents and Denialists

HIV/AIDS 'dissidents' have been compared with Holocaust deniers, to the point where there have been calls for them to be prosecuted in the manner of David Irving, the British historian jailed in Austria in 2006 for maintaining, amongst other problematic points, that there were no gas chambers at Auschwitz (Smyth 2006). The terms AIDS 'dissident' or 'sceptic' cover a broad spectrum of opinion. Dissidents are by no means unified. Different individuals and groups have made various claims about the nature of HIV, the link between HIV and AIDS, and the efficacy of antiretroviral treatments. Some have questioned whether AIDS as a disease exists at all. The majority of dissidents base their theories on what are perceived to be 'holes' in the science underpinning HIV/AIDS 'orthodoxy'. For analysts and policymakers, the question at the heart of the debate is one of censorship. Should dissidents, in the interests of freedom of speech and scientific inquiry, be permitted a platform for their views? After all, in the best traditions of liberalism, and in the spirit of John Stuart Mill (1998), any theory, if 'true', should be able to withstand scrutiny.

The dissident debate may test the boundaries of democratic 'freedoms', but any exercising of this particular 'freedom' would, arguably, have been confined to the margins of the internet and sections of the popular press had it not been for the public statements of Thabo Mbeki – particularly those made between 1999 and 2008, while he was President of South Africa. When Mbeki, leader of a country with one of the highest rates of HIV/AIDS in the world, announced his 'scepticism' concerning the causal link between HIV and AIDS in 1999, the world reacted with incredulity. Mbeki pointed to the inequity of Northern pharmaceutical monopolies and the socio-political construction of an unchallengeable scientific consensus that bore little reality to the

African experience. The backlash was immediate and vociferous. Indeed, if Mbeki is known for anything outside the confines of African politics, it is as the statesman who queried the existence of HIV/AIDS. Although he publicly recanted many of his more extreme views on the matter, his name has been forever smeared, particularly in the developed world. At the same time, Mbeki was not the only African leader to express doubts over the validity of established 'AIDS orthodoxy'. Namibian President Sam Nujoma and Kenyan Nobel Laureate Wangari Maathai entered the debate, both expressing concerns that the disease was laboratory-concocted by agents of Western governments.

From a policymaking perspective, it is critical to take into account the impact of the dissident stance in shaping political and social responses to HIV/AIDS. This chapter considers two specific issues relating to the dissident debate: it outlines the development and evolution of the sceptics' case against the so-called HIV/AIDS orthodoxy and evaluates their claims that they have been unfairly marginalized by the scientific community. It then assesses the dissenter perspective in terms of its potential for harm, and considers whether this necessitates a curtailment of the dissenters' right to disseminate their views.

Questioning scientific 'dogma'

Are the perspectives of AIDS sceptics dangerous? As with climate sceptics, AIDS sceptics reignited public debate on the nature of scientific enquiry. If there is to be any faith in their validity, scientific theories must be able to withstand scrutiny. Shielding established views from debate is an anathema for most researchers, given the importance of fresh perspectives in advancing knowledge. Harvard academic Jerome Kagan (2009) has outlined the importance of 'opposition' to orthodoxy:

> Every democracy requires an opposition party to prevent one temporarily in power from becoming despotic. And every society needs a cohort of intellectuals to check the dominance of a single perspective when its ideological hand becomes too heavy. The first cohort of natural scientists, especially Kepler, Galileo, Bacon, and Newton, assumed this responsibility when Christian philosophy dominated European thought and their work catalyzed the Enlightenment.

Copernicus and Galileo are famous precisely because their work represented such profound threats to existing orthodoxies. In turn, Einstein is famous because of the questions his work provoked regarding the validity of Newtonian physics. That he challenged successfully the pervading paradigm, resulted in significant advances in the field of theoretical physics. On this basis, the dissident lobby, if it is not necessarily to be embraced, should at least be tolerated.

The general contemporary perception of 'science' is one of neutrality; unlike the 'social sciences', 'hard' science is seen to be based on fact, driven by the rigorous testing of hypotheses by highly-trained, impartial observers.[1] In this way, so the understanding goes, the 'truth' about a given phenomena can be ascertained. This view of science remains based largely on Sir Francis Bacon's prescriptions from 1620. As Bacon put it, 'science proceeds through the collection of observations without prejudice' (cited in Goodstein 2000). However, the reality of what constitutes 'good science' is more complex. 'Facts' themselves are problematic. The commonly held view of facts tends to coalesce around three key points: 1) facts are made known to unbiased observers *via* the senses 2) facts are generated prior to and independent of theory 3) facts form a firm and reliable foundation for knowledge (Chalmers 1999). However, problems arise because, in order to be understood, facts need to be interpreted. Furthermore, observers need to be taught to analyse and interpret the facts. For example, a doctor needs to be trained to read an x-ray. In the same way, scientists need to be trained to interpret the results of their experiments – and 'facts', of course, can change. Before Copernicus and Galileo, Europe held geocentrism to be 'fact'. Observations are frequently distorted by what the researcher expects to see. Judgements on the truth of observations depend largely on what is already assumed or 'known' (Chalmers 1999). At the same time, mass observation of the same phenomena generally results in a consensus. Galileo's theories and observations survived because, despite being thoroughly tested, they remained consistent. That being said, simply because a theory has passed all the tests to which it has been subjected, does not mean this will always be the case. Any long-accepted paradigm – Newtonian physics for instance, which in turn displaced Aristotelian physics – can be rendered rapidly obsolete by new developments in the field, in this case, Einstein's work on gravity. Copernicus and Galileo remain the template for scientific revolution: question everything. As Galileo himself put it, 'in matters of science the authority of thousands is not worth the humble reasoning of one single person' (Galileo cited in Goodstein 2000).

'Falsification' is a theory of science that accepts that observation is guided by theory and that no single theory is ever 'true'. Rather, prevailing theories are simply the best available at the time (Chalmers 1999).

Science thus progresses and evolves through a system of trial and error, as a never-ending cycle of theory and experimentation (Crowell 1998). A good scientific theory is one that is 'falsifiable'. That is, it must be able to be tested. A theory that cannot be tested is of limited value. If a scientist argues that all metals expand when heated, then this claim can be readily tested. It is important, then, that science stay fresh, that scientists continuously propose hypotheses and attempt to falsify them. Karl Popper, the eminent twentieth-century philosopher of science, a key exponent of this view, argued that bold theories are imperative, even if they turn out to be wrong, because we learn and develop from our mistakes (Keuth 2005). The Austrian philosopher, Paul Feyerabend, argued that there is only one principle of scientific method and that is 'that anything goes' (Chalmers 1999). The role of the maverick, paradigm-questioning scientist is thus arguably one of noble pedigree; a heritage to which many of the dissidents have attempted to lay claim.

The dissidents and their views

There are a number of prominent AIDS dissidents, some of whom have been successful in communicating their views to the wider public *via* the popular press. As Nicoli Nattrass (2010) demonstrates in her provocatively-titled article 'Still Crazy After All These Years', despite notable advances in the study of HIV/AIDS since the 1980s, many of the dissidents continue to cling to their claims. Notable dissidents include American journalist Celia Farber, who has published in mainstream titles like *Spin* (1989, 1991, 1993, 1996, and 1997), *Mothering* (1998), *Gear* (2000), *Harper's Magazine* (2006a), and British journalist Neville Hodgkinson, who published numerous articles in the *Sunday Times* between 1992 and 1994. The so-called 'Perth Group', fronted by the Greek-born biophysicist Eleni Papadopulos-Eleopulos, has published extensively on HIV/AIDS. Two of its members were invited to sit on Thabo Mbeki's 'Presidential Advisory Panel' in 2000. A relatively new entrant into the fray has been the Canadian academic Rebecca Culshaw (2007), a 'mathematical biologist' and author of *Science Sold Out: Does HIV Really Cause AIDS?* However, by far-and-away the most prominent of the dissidents is Peter Duesberg, tenured professor of molecular and cell biology at the University of California, Berkeley. He was elected to the US National Academy of Sciences in 1986 and is the one-time recipient of an Outstanding Investigator Grant from the US National Institutes of Health. A cancer specialist, in 1987 he produced a paper entitled 'Retroviruses as Carcinogens and Pathogens: Expectations and Reality' in which he questioned the harmfulness of HIV, arguing that the 'virus is not sufficient to cause AIDS and that there is no evidence, besides its presence in a latent form, that it is necessary for AIDS' (Duesberg 1987). In a short paper the following year, published in *Science*, Duesberg (1988) posited that 'the human immuno-deficiency virus (HIV) is not the cause of AIDS' because researchers have failed to demonstrate conclusively that the micro-organism is the causative agent of AIDS. He argued that HIV is 'biochemically inactive and harmless' and that AIDS does not behave as a contagious disease (http://www.duesberg.com). According to his staunchest advocates, Celia Farber (2006a, 2006b) and his biographer, Harvey Bialy (2004), another American molecular biologist, Duesberg has been pilloried for daring to question received wisdom and has, as a result, seen his academic reputation destroyed in a malicious witch-hunt. Farber (2006a) argues that Duesberg, having previously found generous sources of funding for his work, subsequently found his grant applications rejected at every turn. The University of California, Berkeley attempted to force him out and there are claims, listed on Duesberg's website,[2] that the Clinton White House made an effort, in 1996, to bribe him into a retraction of his views. Farber (2006b) recounts Duesberg's tribulations in some detail in her book, *Serious Adverse Events*. What makes Duesberg stand out from amongst the other dissenters is that, prior to his foray into the HIV/AIDS debate, he was an eminently respected scientist, as his election to the National Academy of Sciences attests. It is for this reason that he is cited heavily by those in the dissident community and so actively loathed by those like the American biomedical researcher Robert Gallo (Gallo *et al* 2006), the 'co-discoverer' of HIV and a 'founding father' of the 'AIDS orthodoxy'.

It would be an oversimplification to present the dissident group as having any unified position on the nature of HIV/AIDS. Views differ considerably; here are some of the arguments:

- HIV has not been shown to exist as a unique, exogenously-acquired retrovirus (Perth Group)
- It has not been demonstrated that AIDS is sexually transmitted (Perth Group)
- HIV exists but is harmless (Peter Duesberg)
- AIDS is caused by drug abuse (Peter Duesberg)
- AIDS is not a disease but a 'socio-political construct' (Rebecca Culshaw)
- HIV/AIDS drugs are toxic and do more harm than good (Anthony Brink, Celia Farber, Thabo Mbeki, David Rasnick, Perth Group)
- an AIDS 'industry' has evolved that is both racist and exploitative (Mbeki)

- AIDS was created as a biological weapon by agents of the apartheid regime or was created by the CIA to exterminate Africans (Wolff Geisler, Wangari Maathai).

Collectively, the chief criticisms levelled against the dissenters are those of either poor scholarship or lack of specialist knowledge, or both. In many respects, especially with regard to 'popular' authors like Celia Farber and Rebecca Culshaw, the charge of poor scholarship stands. Farber's *Serious Adverse Events* is largely devoid of references. Statistics are quoted, assertions made, and science dismissed with little attempt to provide evidence. Farber's 2006a piece, 'Out of Control: AIDS and the Corruption of Medical Science' in *Harper's Magazine* prompted a detailed rebuttal from, amongst others, Robert Gallo, who accused her of 'using a plethora of false, misleading, biased and unfair statements' (Gallo *et al* 2006). Faber makes bold pronouncements: for instance, the contention that pregnancy can result in potential 'false positives' being recorded in HIV tests, without providing any references for such an assertion. However, the main charge levelled against Farber by Gallo *et al* (2006) is that she is not a scientist and that she is 'clearly out of her depth'. Culshaw, however, ranks as an academic. She was assistant professor of mathematics at the University of Texas at Tyler in 2006 when she wrote *Science Sold Out*, and has carried out research on the mathematical modelling of the interaction of HIV with the immune system. However, despite her academic credentials, Culshaw's work, too, lacks references. She even fails to acknowledge those in the dissident community to whom she is clearly intellectually indebted. Ken Witwer (2007), a member of AIDSTruth, a group established in 2006 to rebut dissident claims, has produced a refutation almost comparable in length to Culshaw's 100-page text. Witwer argues that it is incredible that a 'serious' academic sees fit to draw the majority of her material from largely non-peer-reviewed work. Culshaw also relies heavily and frequently on Farber, whose work, we have already established, does not conform to academic standards.

From the dissident perspective, a lack of formal academic qualifications is not necessarily viewed as an obstacle. In a speech to the Conference on Science and Democracy in Naples in 2001, Anthony Liversidge (2001), a one-time journalist for the now defunct Science Fiction publication *OMNI* and a supporter of Peter Duesberg, expressed his credentials in the field of AIDS research as follows; 'I have devoted a large amount of time to researching, thinking and writing about the topic, and have interviewed a wide range of people with different perspectives in the field. So while I am not academically qualified in the specific field of retroviruses, my view is informed by personal dealings with its leading figures and their arguments ... And to cite another credential, I do not have a personal axe to grind. I have no direct career involvement within science or medicine'. As will be argued below, Liversidge is not alone in venturing beyond his area of expertise.

What of the dissident scientists and researchers? On the face of it, some sport impressive credentials. Kary Mullis, for instance, who holds a PhD from the University of California, Berkeley, won the Nobel Prize for chemistry in 1993. However, closer inspection of certain key individuals' qualifications serves to undermine their positions on HIV/AIDS. The 'Perth Group', founded in 1981 in Perth, Western Australia, is headed by 'Dr' Eleni Papadopulos-Eleopulos. On dissident websites like 'virusmyth', she is listed as having a PhD and is also, on occasion, afforded the title of 'Professor' (virusmyth.com). On the Perth Group's own webpage, press interviews have been published in which Papadopulos-Eleopulos is described as a biophysicist and afforded the title of 'Doctor' (Johnson 1997). In reality, she holds an undergraduate degree in physics from a Romanian university and, at the time of the 1997 interview referred to above, was employed as a medical technician in the Royal Perth Hospital (AIDSTruth 2008). She and fellow members of the Perth Group conduct their HIV/ AIDS research in what they acknowledge to be their 'spare time'. They are not affiliated to any academic or medical institution. In a terse response to an attack on her credibility by Professor John Moore (2006), a professor of microbiology and immunology at the Weill Medical College of Cornell University, at the XVI International AIDS Conference, Papadopulos-Eleopulos (2006) argued that 'the value of a theory or any other work cannot be judged on the basis of whatever academic credentials or lack of them the person has'. However, when she was called as an expert witness for the defence in the Australian case of Andre Chad Parenzee, an HIV-positive individual accused of endangering others by engaging in unprotected sex, the presiding judge ruled that:

Ms Papadopulos-Eleopulos has no formal qualifications in medicine, biology, virology, immunology, epidemiology or any other medical disciplines. She has never treated or been directly involved in clinical trials of any kind relating to any disease. Her duties at the Royal Perth Hospital are to test people for sensitivity to ultraviolet radiation.

Ms Papadopulos-Eleopulos claims that she conducts research in the area of HIV/AIDS in her private time. It became clear that, when she spoke about research, she meant reading various medical papers about the research of others. Her experience with the HIV virus and with AIDS is limited to reading and critiquing the work of researchers involved in various studies. She purports to have expertise to speak on the subject of virology, epidemiology, electron microscopy, biology and immunology. She has no practical experience in any of these areas. She has no formal qualifications in these disciplines (Supreme Court of Southern Australia 2007).

Tellingly, none of the dissident scientists, according to their critics, are actually actively engaged in HIV/AIDS research or publishing their results in peer-reviewed journals. Like Papadopulos-Eleopulos, the majority developed their theories second-hand, using and interpreting other people's data. In her defense against this very accusation, that 'denialists don't publish any of their own work. They simply criticize, ignorantly, the work of scientists who do', Papadopulos-Eleopulos (2006) offered this rebuttal:

> our publications contain a lot of original ideas and work. Although it is not necessary for us to perform experiments based on our ideas, we would have preferred to do them. However, due to lack of funds we have been unable to perform our original experiments. Science has progressed on the basis of new ideas and theories being presented many times by either one person or a group of people and then experiments being carried out by either another person or group of people. In fact, some of the most important progressions in science were based on ideas of people who never performed the experiments themselves.

For the dissidents, inability, through lack of funding, to conduct original research is evidence of a wider conspiracy by vested interests like the pharmaceutical industry to prevent the HIV/AIDS orthodoxy from being challenged. Farber (2006b) argues that during the 1970s and 1980s, Duesberg rarely struggled to secure funding. She states that 'prior to 1987, he was one of the most generously funded scientists in the nation and had never had a grant turned down. Since 1987, he has submitted a total of twenty-three grant proposals ... and every single one has been rejected'. Duesberg himself argues on his website homepage that his findings 'have been a thorn in the side of the medical establishment and drug companies since 1987. Instead of engaging in scientific debate, however, the only response has been to cut off funding' (http://www.duesberg.com). Journalist Anthony Liversidge (1995) likewise, in an article for

The Cultural Studies Times, a free paper offered by Routledge, empathized, 'Peter Duesberg is virtually without grants, graduate students or influence, prevented from replying to his critics in leading journals and routinely ignored or detracted in the mainstream press. The Nobel Prize he was expected to win for his earlier work has gone to others, and coverage of his ideas in the science news journals and in the mainstream press has been fitful, gratuitously antagonistic and uniformly disparaging of the heresy and heretic both'.

A case for censorship?

The 'passion of Peter Duesberg' (Farber 2006b) and the wider dissident debate might have remained confined largely to the peripheries of the internet – the dissidents having largely failed to convince the world of their cause – if it had not been for the 'conversion' of the then South African President, Thabo Mbeki in 1999. In an open letter to 'world leaders' in April 2000, published in the *Washington Post*, he articulated his view of an entrenched 'AIDS industry' and an unassailable orthodoxy:

> I am convinced that our urgent task is to respond to the specific threat that faces us as Africans. We will not eschew this obligation in favour of the comfort of the recitation of a catechism that may very well be a correct response to the specific manifestation of AIDS in the West. We will not, ourselves, condemn our own people to death by giving up the search for specific and targeted responses to the specifically African incidence of HIV-AIDS. I make these comments because our search for these specific and targeted responses is being stridently condemned by some in our country and the rest of the world as constituting a criminal abandonment of the fight against HIV-AIDS. Some elements of this orchestrated campaign of condemnation worry me very deeply. It is suggested, for instance, that there are some scientists who are 'dangerous and discredited' with whom nobody, including ourselves, should communicate or interact. In an earlier period in human history, these would be heretics that would be burnt at the stake! Not long ago, in our own country, people were killed, tortured, imprisoned and prohibited from being quoted in private and in public because the established authority believed that their views were dangerous and discredited. We are now being asked to do precisely the same thing that the racist apartheid tyranny we opposed did, because, it is said, there

exists a scientific view that is supported by the majority, against which dissent is prohibited (Mbeki 2000a).

As the freely-elected leader of a country with one of the highest rates of HIV/AIDS prevalence in the world (and, moreover, the successor of Nelson Mandela, architect of South Africa's largely bloodless transition from apartheid police state to democracy and arguably one of the most respected people alive), Mbeki's views could not be viewed purely within the context of freedom of expression or academic curiosity. Through the auspices of his Presidential Advisory Panel, convened in May 2000, Mbeki went on to facilitate the communication of the views of dissidents including Peter Duesberg and the Perth Group to a far greater audience than they could previously have hoped to command.

Was Mbeki, in his position as leading African statesman, entitled to express publicly his dissident sympathies and, indeed, did his stance cause 'harm'? Parallels between the AIDS dissidents and holocaust deniers like David Irving abound in the popular print and electronic media. In the electronic *First Post*, A. S. H. Smyth (2006) demands that 'if Holocaust-deniers deserve to be punished, so do AIDS-deniers. It is high time African governments outlawed denial of the epidemic, and prosecuted those who perpetuate misinformation about AIDS or in any way undermine efforts to tackle it'. Gallo *et al* (2006), in their response to Celia Farber's *Harper's Magazine* article, posted on activist websites like the AIDS Education Global Information System (AEGIS) and the Treatment Action Campaign (TAC), argue:

> As with Holocaust denialism, AIDS denialism is pseudo-scientific and contradicts an immense body of research. But in contrast to Holocaust denialism, AIDS denialism directly threatens lives today by trying to fool laypeople at risk of HIV not to get tested for the virus or not to practice safer sex. It also tries to fool those who need ARVs not to take them.

The 'right-to-reply' has presented numerous editors of both scientific and popular publications with a moral dilemma. In the late 1980s and early 1990s, Duesberg (1989, 1991, and 1992) made extensive use of the correspondence pages in the journal *Nature* to ensure that his views on HIV remained centre-stage. The editor, John Maddox (1993) was initially uncomfortable with the idea of censorship: 'what is to be thought of a science journal that publishes attacks on the opinions of a scientist, but which never (or hardly ever) publishes his replies? On the face of things, this is a serious breach of journalistic ethics ... How can such intolerance be justified?' However, Maddox was eventually moved to question Duesberg's right-to-reply in the pages of his journal. He argued, in the pages of *Nature*, that the 'truth is that a person's "right-to-reply" may conflict with a journal's obligation to its readers to provide them with authentic information ... the right of reply must be modulated by its content'. Maddox's subsequent censorship of Duesberg led to accusations of a conspiracy on the part of the scientific community to silence the dissenters (Liversidge 2001).

The trials and tribulations of Galileo, in his battle against the prevailing orthodoxy of his age – geocentrism – have struck a chord with many of the AIDS dissidents, who have referenced widely his struggle against the early seventeenth-century Catholic Church. Peter Duesberg supporter and Nobel Laureate Kary Mullis (1998) argues in his autobiography, *Dancing Naked in the Mind Field*, that 'years from now, people looking back at us will find our acceptance of the HIV theory of AIDS as silly as we find the leaders who excommunicated Galileo. Science as it is practiced today is largely not science at all. What people call science is probably very similar to what was called science in 1634'. Similar examples abound. Anthony Brink (2000), a South African dissident, in the preface to his self-published book *Debating AZT: Mbeki and the AIDS Drug Controversy*, opens with a quotation relating to Galileo's travails with the Church. He goes on to argue that 'concerning my polemical style and sardonic tone, I should explain that I wrote with politicking in mind. (It's a trick I picked up from Galileo. Unable to sell his discovery of the moons of Jupiter to his peers ... he took to pamphleteering the lay public instead)' (Brink 2000). Papadopulos-Eleopulos (2006), likewise, cites Galileo as an inspiration 'We should never forget Galileo being put before the inquisition [*sic*]. It would be even worse if we allowed scientific orthodoxy to become the inquisition'. Anthony Liversidge (2001) also argues that 'science still frequently imitates the Roman Catholic Church at the time of Galileo. What should be intellectual debate becomes a bitter power struggle'.

Defining the motivation for the dissident movement is difficult. In part, this is because the denialists represent a broad church and one that is often far from unified. As Papadopulos-Eleopulos (2006) admits, the Perth Group clashed with Duesberg over the existence of HIV in the mid-1990s. With other high profile dissident debates, like that of climate change, a political motive is usually clear. Prominent climate change sceptics like Princeton physicist Professor William Happer, who addressed the US Senate Committee on Environment and Public Works on anthropogenic influences on global temperature change in February 2009, tend to have links to conservative advocacy groups. Happer, for example, chairs the right-wing think tank the George C Marshall Institute, which has, in turn, accepted donations from Exxon-Mobil in order to conduct research into, amongst other issues, climate change (Carey 2006). The International Conference on Climate Change, held in New York City in March 2009, brought together leading climate sceptics from around the world. Attendees included representatives from right-wing think tanks like the Heartland Institute, the Ayn Rand Institute, the Carbon Sense Coalition and the Committee for a Constructive Tomorrow, some of which have in the past also received funding from Exxon-Mobil (Revkin 2009). The point is that the doubts of many climate change sceptics form just one aspect of their wider conservative political agendas. It is difficult to say the same for the AIDS dissidents. Peter Duesberg's (1996) book, *Inventing the AIDS Virus* was published by Regnery, a well known publisher of right-wing material, and Culshaw's work has been hosted on libertarian websites like LewRockwell.com (http://www.lewrockwell. com). However, it is difficult to afford the dissidents a political profile other than that of their stated belief in free speech and an urge to be viewed as Galileo-style mavericks. Unlike climate scepticism, which converges with the interests of the petrochemical and energy industries and is thus frequently well funded, AIDS denialism is largely financially unproductive. Duesberg and the Perth Group have been effectively reduced to begging on their websites (http://www.duesberg.com and http://www.theperthgroup.com).

AIDS denialists appear to have a great deal in common with conspiracy theorists generally, exhibiting a basic mistrust of authority, both medical and political. They tend to view themselves as 'truth-seekers' rather than denialists (Kalichman 2009). Moreover, when analysed in conjunction with other conspiracy theorists, like those preoccupied with the alternative 'truths' relating to the Holocaust, 9/11, the moon landings, and UFOs, the language and methods of the dissidents become indistinguishable from the rest (arguably, some climate change sceptics meet the criteria for 'conspiracy theorists' too). All such groups start from a predetermined position that is then duly defended against all-comers. Similarly, evidence is cherry-picked and quoted out of context, and 'evil forces' (in the case of HIV, pharmaceutical companies) are deemed to be manipulating the public, creating a 'false reality' (Kalichman 2009). Conspiracy theorists also veer towards paranoia and see 'evidence' of persecution in unlikely places. The Perth Group, for example, notes as evidence of a conspiracy by the scientific community to silence them all of their papers that have failed to pass the peer-review process demanded by mainstream academic publishers (http://www.the-perthgroup.com). Duesberg perceives his inability to secure funding as proof of a plot to silence him. The reality is that mainstream science, rather than trying to crush the dissidents, would prefer to ignore them. Thabo Mbeki, however, made the implementation of this latter strategy rather more problematic.

Opposing AIDS dissenters has proven difficult because freedom of speech is a cornerstone of any democratic state. From Voltaire's 'I do not agree with what you have to say, but I'll defend to the death your right to say it' to John Stuart Mill's (1998) injunction that

> if all mankind minus one, were of one opinion, and only one person were of the contrary opinion, mankind would be no more justified in silencing that one person, than he, if he had the power, would be justified in silencing mankind ... the peculiar evil of silencing the expression of opinion is, that it is robbing the human race; posterity as well as the existing generation; those who dissent from the opinion, still more than those who hold it.

It is thus unsurprising that when a complaint was lodged about a dissident segment on a South African talk-radio slot, aired in April 2005, the Broadcasting Complaints Commission of South Africa ruled that 'the nature of freedom of expression is that we should not, and cannot, stop people from disseminating their ideas ... Let the listeners decide for themselves' (cited in Geffen 2007).

Here it is necessary to return to the question of 'free speech' and 'harm'. Dissidents make frequent reference to the dangers of censorship in restricting scientific debate. However, even in the most liberal societies, free speech generally has its limits. John Stuart Mill (1998), in *On Liberty*, argued that individual freedom could be justly curtailed if it caused harm. Nathan Geffen (2007), a high profile member of the South African AIDS-activist group the Treatment Action Campaign, points out that many democracies have laws against hate speech, certain forms of pornography, libel, and certain extremist political symbols (Nazi regalia in Germany, for instance). It is arguably possible to equate certain forms of AIDS dissent with public endangerment – for example, if such material encourages individuals to abandon their treatment programmes – the equivalent of shouting 'fire' in a crowded cinema (Kalichman 2009). In such instances, then, the issue is about public health rather than freedom of expression. In South Africa, the 'public health' factor is clear;

evidence suggests that under Mbeki a significant proportion of the population came to doubt the AIDS orthodoxy. A Harvard University study conducted in 2004 found that 48 percent of black South Africans believed that the ANC government had taken a sensible line on HIV/AIDS (Wang 2008).

Thabo Mbeki's right to dissent

Mbeki's questioning of the 'HIV/AIDS-hypothesis' ensured both the elevation of the dissident debate to the front pages of the popular media and his immediate vilification across the globe. Controversial announcements emanating from the offices of Mbeki and his health minister, the medical doctor Manto Tshabalala-Msimang (1999–2008), prompted international disbelief and outrage in almost equal measure. In a now-famous speech to community groups in Soweto, Dr Tshabalala-Msimang (2004) stressed that the

> use of alternative remedies such as garlic, lemon and ginger for chronically ill patients is very important. We should eat garlic because of its antibacterial and anti-fungal properties, lemon because of Vitamin C and olive oil as a source of Vitamin A and E. All these vitamins are good antioxidants and they are good for maintaining optimal health.

In outlining the government's efforts to improve the health of those living with HIV/AIDS, she did not once refer to ARVs. She also strongly promoted the consumption of beetroot and the African potato as natural remedies in the fight against HIV/AIDS. Her insistence on the healing properties of the above foodstuffs spawned two of her more polite nicknames; 'Dr Garlic' and 'Dr Beetroot'. Much was made of pronouncements like this one, made during the course of a 2005 press conference: 'raw garlic and a skin of the lemon – not only do they give you a beautiful face and skin but they also protect you from disease' (cited in Paroske 2009). The Treatment Action Campaign referred to her as a 'murderer' and, in March 2003, attempted to file manslaughter charges against her for causing the unnecessary deaths of thousands of South Africans. Mbeki himself, post-2000, in an effort to diffuse the furore created by his denialism, ceased to make public pronouncements on HIV/AIDS, although he continued to allow Tshabalala-Msimang to operate as the government's 'AIDS tsar'. However, in August 2007, Mbeki's views were once again brought under the spotlight when he dismissed his popular deputy health minister, Nozizwe Madlala-Routledge, who had overseen the government's rollout of ARVs, for attending an AIDS summit without his permission (Nattrass 2008). The decision to dismiss her was viewed by AIDS activists as symptomatic of Mbeki demonstrating his support for the returning Tshabalala-Msimang, who had been off work for nine months following a liver transplant (Tshabalala-Msimang died as a result of complications in 2009).

Mbeki's leadership stance on HIV/AIDS may be difficult for critics to comprehend. Yet there is arguably more to his stance than the pseudo-intellectualism of which he has been accused. Joy Wang (2008) argues persuasively that the best way to understand Mbeki's denialism is to view it as a struggle against neo-colonialism. What Mbeki reacted to most vociferously in the AIDS debate was what he perceived to be the dehumanization and demonization of Africans by the West. He contested the implication that African culture – and particularly African male culture – is to blame for the spread of HIV/AIDS. In 2002, an anonymous pamphlet widely believed (Wang 2008) to have been authored by Mbeki, entitled 'Castro Hlongwane, Caravans, Cats, Geese, Foot & Mouth and Statistics: HIV/AIDS and the Struggle for the Humanisation of the African', was distributed extensively *via* ANC offices. The pamphlet railed against both the greed of the major multinational pharmaceutical companies and the racism inherent in much of the AIDS discourse (Anonymous 2002). The author quotes journalist Charlene Smith, writing in the *Washington Post* in 2000, as typifying the racialized nature of the debate: 'Here (in Africa), (AIDS) is spread primarily by heterosexual sex – spurred by men's attitudes towards women. We won't end this epidemic until we understand the role of tradition and religion – and of a culture in which rape is endemic and has become a prime means of transmitting disease, to young women as well as children'. In certain respects, Mbeki's position is entirely reasonable: an attempt to shift the blame for the pandemic from the purported 'iniquities' of Africans themselves to a global system that perpetuates the spread of HIV/AIDS by ensuring that Africans continue to live in poverty.

The harm principle

Thus far, the arguments presented hinge on the issue of harm. If Mbeki's view can be demonstrated to have led to loss of life, then his belief system moves beyond being one of personal conscience and into the realms of more emotive territory – at minimum, gross irresponsibility. What makes Mbeki's scepticism so difficult for AIDS activists is that

South Africa has witnessed a 'lost decade' in the fight against the pandemic. ANC documents from 1994 make it plain that the party was aware of the HIV/AIDS threat and even produced accurate estimates predicting its spread if left unchecked (Heywood 2004). However, in 1999, after absorbing many of the dissidents' arguments, Mbeki began proselytizing their views within his party. It was during this time that the newly-established and increasingly vocal Treatment Action Campaign (TAC) began to demand AZT, an antiretroviral effective in reducing significantly the risk of mother-to-child transmission, for pregnant women with HIV. In a parliamentary speech in October 1999, Mbeki for the first time questioned publicly the safety of AZT. Later that year, seemingly in response to ever-more strident calls from civil society groups like the TAC, the government, still stalling on committing itself to any ARV programme, demanded instead that the South African Medicines Control Council (MCC) conduct a safety assessment of AZT. Mbeki accused the TAC of being a front for the major pharmaceutical companies, and thus an agent of imperialism (an unlikely situation given the TAC's active participation in the infamous court case brought by the major pharmaceutical companies against the South African government's plans to expand access to generic drugs – Chapter 8) (Heywood 2004). Countrywide distribution of AZT was stalled for four years, despite the MCC during that time twice ruling that the drug's benefits outweighed its side effects. The government finally acquiesced to pressure only after an instruction from the South African Constitutional Court in 2002 (Nattrass 2006). Tshabalala-Msimang, as Minister of Health, delayed the rollout of AZT to people living with AIDS until, with the 2004 general election fast approaching and the government under international scrutiny, a cabinet revolt in August 2003 forced a change in policy (Johnson 2009). While Tshabalala-Msimang accepted the cabinet's decision, her department was exceedingly slow in implementing the policy, failing to hit its stated target of having 50,000 people on treatment by the end of the first year of the programme. There is also evidence that the Minister personally referred sufferers to 'traditional' healers (Chapter 5), some of whom treated the disease with concoctions made from 'supermarket ingredients' (Nattrass 2006). Tshabalala-Msimang courted further controversy by actively supporting entrepreneurial vitamin salesman Matthias Rath, whose Rath Health Foundation has promoted expensive courses of vitamins as a more effective solution to fighting HIV than, as he put it, 'toxic' drugs like AZT (Geffen 2005). A South African High Court ruling in June 2008 banned Rath from advertising his product as a cure for AIDS.

The impact of Mbeki's views on HIV/AIDS (alongside those of Tshabalala-Msimang) in quantifiable terms, became apparent in two studies, the first published in the journal *AIDS* in 2006 and the second in the *Journal of Acquired Immune Deficiency Syndrome* in 2008. The authors of the first study, Chopra *et al* (2006), found that awareness of ARVs amongst the general public in South Africa was surprising low. Many South Africans perceived ARVs as simply one treatment amongst a range of options. Almost half of the respondents on ARVs reported using traditional and alternative remedies before switching to prescribed drugs (Chapter 5). The study concluded that 'if antiretroviral agents are to compete more successfully in the therapeutic continuum, there needs to be explicit recognition of, and further strategies to counter, the attraction of alternative therapies for patients and the systematic promotion these treatments receive' (Chopra *et al* 2006). In the second study, researchers from the Harvard School of Public Health attempted to ascertain the human cost of delaying the rollout of ARVs in South Africa between 2000 and 2005. They compared the number of people who actually received ARV treatment during this period with the numbers who might have received it, taking into account South Africa's circumstances at the time. The study suggested that 'more than 330,000 lives or approximately 2.2 million person years were lost because a feasible and timely ARV treatment program was not implemented in South Africa' (Chigwedere *et al* 2008). The Harvard researchers estimated that during this period 35,000 babies acquired HIV *via* mother-to-child transmission, something that might have been averted through the administration of the ARV Nevirapine (Chigwedere *et al* 2008). In this respect, Mbeki's public position has, literally, cost lives.

Conclusion

For much of the late 1980s and early 1990s, the dissident debate remained largely confined to the margins of the internet. However, where South Africa was concerned, Thabo Mbeki's increasing acceptance of the dissidents' arguments ensured that once obscure and ridiculed theories now formed the guiding principles for a head of state charged with containing his country's HIV/AIDS pandemic. Despite 'removing' himself from the dissident debate in 2000, his proxy, Health Minister Manto Tshabalala-Msimang, continued, until the end of the Mbeki administration in 2008, to ensure that dissident views remained a crucial influence on the government's response to HIV/AIDS. The fact that activists were required to drag the government before the Constitutional Court in order to ensure the provision of ARVs for HIV-infected women demonstrates the extent to which the debate transcended the political issues of freedom of speech and resistance to perceived neo-imperialism. It is possible to argue that, whatever their intentions, Mbeki and Tshabalala-Msimang's public stance generated a significant level of public scepticism regarding HIV/AIDS. The legacy of overt AIDS scepticism in elite circles has been a culture of complacency and confusion amongst non-elites. If projections are accurate, hundreds of thousands of lives have been lost unnecessarily (Chigwedere *et al* 2008). South African AIDS policymaking has been driven by what is largely an internet conspiracy theory. While it is possible to evaluate Mbeki's position in terms of a perceived neo-colonial struggle, or even as an attempt to highlight the extent to which poverty and HIV/AIDS go hand-in-hand, it is nonetheless difficult to excuse the ANC government's record on HIV/AIDS and the missed opportunities their policies represent. While South Africa is the most obvious case in which the sceptical attitude of political elites had a profound and negative impact on policy and governance, the fact remains that many African elites, whilst not dissidents, have been relatively ambivalent with respect to addressing HIV/AIDS. Health spending as a proportion of GDP remains low (Chapter 1) and political will to fight the pandemic is often lacking. The views of political elites, as much as the efficacy of drugs and condoms, are central to arresting the spread of HIV/AIDS in Africa.

5
Traditional Medicine and the Politics of the 'Witchcraft Paradigm'

For the past 30 years, healthcare practitioners around the world, both traditional and biomedical, have had to come to terms with the day-to-day realities of treating HIV and AIDS. In many African countries, a significant proportion of the responsibility has fallen to practitioners of traditional medicine; there is an often-quoted figure that suggests that up to 80 percent of the sub-Saharan population consults traditional healers and makes use of traditional medicine for their primary healthcare needs (see for example WHO 2002, 2008b). The international media spotlight has fallen on the tendency of African traditional practitioners to classify HIV/AIDS sufferers as 'bewitched' or contaminated with 'pollutants'. Behind the headlines lie a number of representations of illness and affliction that are distinctly African, and frequently at odds with 'orthodox' 'Western' ideas of disease. Where the language of 'pollution' is concerned, there are distinct parallels between African perspectives on contamination of the body and worldwide concerns about contamination of the environment. However, in a purely medical sense, the 'pollution' designation runs contrary to prevailing 'Western' perspectives on the diagnosis of disease. It is crucial that more attention be paid by governments, donor agencies and NGOs to working with, and through, traditional African cosmologies. This chapter outlines some of the main elements common to many African cultures' understanding of illness and its causality, and highlights the difficulties that this paradigm represents for 'orthodox' disease prevention and treatment programmes. In addition, it considers the attempts by African governments to reconcile the tensions caused by competing worldviews on disease with respect to HIV/AIDS treatment and prevention.

At present, the life expectancy of HIV/AIDS sufferers hinges on their access to ARVs. ARV distribution is therefore a vital aspect of HIV/AIDS management. The success of programmes like PEPFAR (Chapter 6) in increasing ARV accessibility has meant an improvement in the lives of millions of sufferers. However, it is neither drug availability nor price (Chapter 8) that guarantees effective treatment; it is also necessary for people to have faith in the treatment on offer. Biomedicine complies with an Enlightenment model of disease management that has 'rational' science at its core – and the veracity of 'rational' science goes largely unquestioned in Europe and North America. For instance, data gathered in 2005, show that 69 percent of the British public believe that scientists 'tell the truth' (Worcester 2006). In the West, then, while interest in traditional medicines is growing (WHO 2002), a centuries-old history of trust in scientific 'truth' means that there is relatively little concern regarding the efficacy of biomedicine. Confidence in the latest HIV/AIDS treatments is relatively assured. This Western worldview is by no means universal, which, with respect to the biomedical management of HIV/AIDS in Africa has created significant challenges for prevention and treatment programmes.

A community's conceptualization of disease forms part of its cosmology, or indigenous knowledge system (IKS). The Centre for Indigenous Knowledge Systems (CEFIKS) defines the IKS concept as:

> the complex set of knowledge and technologies existing and developed around specific conditions of populations and communities indigenous to a particular geographic area. It is the knowledge that people in a given community have developed over time, and continue to develop. Much of the knowledge is passed down from generation to generation, usually by word of mouth (CEFIKS 2009).

Peoples' perceptions of the mechanics of disease, how they become ill, why they become ill and how illness should be combated, are pivotal in determining how they react to illness, how they might seek to prevent it and with what manner of healthcare system they engage in order to treat it. Simply put, it is likely that those beholden to a non-Western illness identity will tend to gravitate towards non-Western forms of treatment. China is a case in point. Up to 50 percent of Chinese medical consumption consists of traditional remedies. In Malaysia, too, more is spent annually on traditional medicine than allopathic remedies (WHO 2002). Likewise, South Korea and Vietnam have highly developed traditional medical sectors (WHO 2006c). The origins and reliability of current estimates of the precise extent of African reliance on traditional medicine have been queried (Ashforth 2005), but there is no doubt that traditional healers play an important role in the lives of many African communities, especially in rural areas where 'Western' doctors might be unavailable. In countries like Uganda, the traditional healer-to-population ratio ranges between 1:200 and 1:400 – compared to the biomedical practitioner-to-population ratio of 1:20,000 (WHO 2002).

An understanding of African explanations as to how and why diseases spread is thus particularly important for those engaging with the epidemiology of HIV/AIDS across sub-Saharan Africa. While it is impossible to outline a cosmology common to the African continent as a whole, there are, with respect to illness and disease, a number of common elements that together can be presented as a generalized 'African outlook' on illness identity. International aid and donor agencies (particularly the WHO but more laterally less obvious agencies like the World Bank) have attempted to engage with debates surrounding traditional medicine and traditional healers since the mid-1970s. However, their studies to date have paid little attention to the worldviews on which these 'representations of disease' are based. This is problematic. In many respects, the African cosmology of traditional medicine is potentially dangerous – perhaps nowhere more so than where HIV/AIDS is concerned, given that the concept of communicable diseases sits uncomfortably within this worldview. Preventative programmes based on behavioural change or even risk aversion are of little value if the tenets underlying them are not subscribed to. Ashforth (2001, 2002, 2005) illustrates the dearth of existing analysis in this area and emphasizes how the literature that does, in passing, address belief systems simply tends to note 'that it complicates education programmes'.

Part of the reluctance to engage with this debate is arguably guided by sensitivities concerning cultural relativism. While diversity is, in most respects, something to be celebrated, if the resulting outcomes are negative then the value of such sensitivity must be reassessed. This has been tacitly, although by no means formally, acknowledged: in sub-Saharan Africa, attempts to square traditional beliefs with the mechanics of biomedicine have focused on 're-educating' traditional healers rather than finding ways to accommodate their views. By outlining the traditional African view of disease, this chapter will highlight the problems facing policymakers in their attempts to treat and prevent the spread of HIV/AIDS.

Engaging with traditional medicine

The World Health Organization has a relatively long history of engagement with traditional medicine and traditional healers. In 1976, it produced a paper on 'Traditional Medicine and its Role in the Development of Health Services in Africa' (WHO 1976) for a session of the Regional Committee for Africa. Likewise, the WHO Alma-Ata Declaration of 1978 on Primary Health Care highlighted a role for traditional healers in the provision of healthcare. The WHO's appreciation of the significance of the role of traditional healers in HIV/AIDS management was cemented in 1990, when representatives from the WHO Traditional Medicines Programme, established in 1979 in the wake of Alma-Ata, and the WHO Global Programme on AIDS met in Botswana to consult on ways to expand the role of traditional health practitioners in preventing and controlling HIV/AIDS (WHO 1990). The consultation document argued that:

> Given the paucity of human and material resources available to African governments and the extremely high number of AIDS cases in the region, there is an urgent need to devise new approaches that would contain the further spread of this dread disease ... traditional medicine is part of the health practices of individuals and communities ... governments, therefore, have a responsibility to ensure that traditional medicines are not harmful and to foster what is effective and beneficial, in keeping with the beliefs of the people (WHO 1990).

The WHO (2002) continued to take this direction, stressing the need to engage with traditional healers and traditional medicines, for much of the next decade, putting out a Traditional Medicine Strategy in 2002, in which it called for the greater integration of traditional medicine into national health systems. The Strategy argued that integration would afford allopathic treatments a degree of cultural legitimacy – something that is frequently missing in many parts of the developing world, especially when biomedical diagnoses appear to conflict with established cosmologies and representations of disease and illness. Attempting a universal definition of traditional medicine, the WHO (2002) described it as

> including diverse health practices, approaches, knowledge and beliefs incorporating plant, animal, and/or mineral based medicines, spiritual therapies, manual techniques and exercises applied singularly or in combination to maintain well-being, as well as to treat, diagnose or prevent illness.

This is, obviously, a rather broad description. Approaches to healing and traditional medicine differ markedly across the world, ranging from acupuncture in China, reiki in Japan and ayurvedic yoga in India, to herbal remedies, including aromatherapy, in regions extending throughout Latin America, Africa, Asia and Europe. However, the belief systems on which these approaches are based differ significantly from region to region, making codification and the determination of 'best practice' all but impossible.

Writing for a World Bank publication on Indigenous Knowledge, Edward Green (2004) argued that as orthodox AIDS strategies had to date been largely ineffective in Africa, it was time to consider alternative approaches. He cited the success of Senegal and Uganda in mobilizing traditional healers behind state AIDS strategies and in breaking down barriers between practitioners of biomedical and traditional medicine. The catalyst for Green's proposal was an initiative involving the Ugandan Ministry of Health, the Ugandan National AIDS Commission and a number of NGOs, which in the early 1990s came together to form Traditional and Modern Health Practitioners Together against AIDS (THETA). THETA went on to have some success in encouraging traditional healers to discuss HIV/AIDS with their patients, to promote condom use and to direct their patients to biomedical healthcare providers for testing (UNAIDS 2000b). Similar collaborations have also been attempted in countries including Botswana, the Central African Republic, Malawi, Mozambique, South Africa, Tanzania and Zambia, with varying degrees of success (UNAIDS 2000b). The WHO has also established 'collaborating centres' in Ghana and Mali that study the efficacy of African traditional medicines (WHO 2002). The success of these programmes has been based on the 're-education' of traditional healers and the scientific scrutiny of the efficacy of traditional medicines. Despite the inescapable appeal of integrating traditional healers and traditional medicine within the broader fabric of African healthcare systems, there are arguments for non-integration. Chief amongst them is the seeming incompatibility of traditional and biomedical representations of disease across much of the continent. There are also the arguments that any promotion of traditional medicine might delay or distract people seeking referral for biomedical treatment (UNAIDS 2000b), and that the sanctioning of traditional practitioners might provide a degree of legitimacy for untested medical claims.

Towards an African view of disease

The extent to which African perceptions of disease are 'problematic' or at odds with biomedical practice is central to any discussion on the value of traditional medicine. Broad generalizations about any aspect of 'African culture' and cosmology, including that of disease and illness, can be highly problematic simply due to the sheer size of Africa and the diversity inherent in literally thousands of ethnic and language groups. However, where the representation and understanding of African illness is concerned, certain similarities in worldview across the continent make it possible to think in terms of an African disease paradigm. The super-natural plays a significant role in the African disease paradigm – what Adam Ashforth (2002) has described as a 'witchcraft paradigm'.

Seminal anthropological studies, those by Edward Evans-Pritchard (1937) and Harriett Ngubane (1977) for instance, conducted amongst the Azande of the Central African region and the Zulu of South Africa respectively, highlight a number of commonalities regarding illness and disease, as do similar studies in Tanzania (Beidelman 1963), Uganda (Beattie 1963) and the southern Sudan (Buxton 1963). Similarly, more contem-porary post-AIDS studies, including those by Felicity Thomas (2008), Christine Liddell *et al* (2005), Ashforth (2001, 2002, 2005), Isak Niehaus (2001), Anne Meyer-Weitz *et al* (1998) and Benedicte Ingstad (1990), all point to recurring features common to the cosmologies of many African communities, including an emphasis on the supernatural. Critically, tra-ditional belief systems incorporating elements of the supernatural are by no means confined to rural backwaters; they continue to be prevalent throughout both urban and rural locales. Ashforth's (2005) study of 'witchcraft' in Soweto, a vast, heavily populated former 'township' now officially part of Johannesburg, demonstrates not only that traditional belief systems still dominate in major urban locales, but that they have remained largely impervious to the challenges of 'modernity'.

In Africa, the concepts of illness and healing extend beyond the con-fines of medical practice as it is understood in the West and incorporate an almost religious dimension that is difficult to articulate in English. In Botswana, the fuller meaning of the Setswana word for illness (*bolwetse*) is somewhat lost when translated into English. So is the translation of the term 'healer' (*ngaka*). Likewise, healers themselves are more than simply doctors. They also act as advisors, counsellors, detectives, social workers and, importantly, diviners (Ntloedibe-Kuswani 1999). This is the case for much of sub-Saharan Africa.

The supernatural elements of these African cosmologies become appar-ent when illness is discussed. A significant proportion of African societies separate illnesses into two categories: 'natural' illnesses, and those brought about by some form of malicious human intervention. Death from any-thing other than 'old age' can be perceived to be 'unnatural' (Orubuloye and Oguntimehin 1999). An anthropologist working in the Namibian Caprivi Strip in the early 1960s noted that 'the notion is that all people should grow old and die from old age: if anything happens to them before then it is the result of machinations of evilly disposed persons' (Kruger cited in Thomas 2008).

'Natural' illnesses are those that 'just happen'. As Ngubane's (1977) ground-breaking study of illness in Zulu culture attests, no one is blamed for a 'natural' illness and symptoms are generally treated without recourse to ritual or ceremony (Ngubane 1977). 'Natural' illnesses include colds, influenza, 'childhood diseases' like mumps and measles, and certain forms of mental illness. 'Unnatural' diseases, on the other hand, are those that can result in either sudden death or prolonged illness, like small-pox, chronic dysentery and tuberculosis (Inyang 1986). The existence of 'unnatural' illness forms much of the basis for the 'witchcraft paradigm', which hinges on the idea of responsibility; someone or something is understood to be a catalyst for the visitation of an 'unnatural' illness. As a result, alternative explanations involving malevolent mediums and prox-imate and ultimate causes are usually sought (Liddell *et al* 2005): how was the illness transmitted, and what caused that particular individual to be affected by the illness? Across much of Africa, illnesses of this nature are usually understood to be caused by 'pollutants', often deliberately placed to contaminate the victim unknowingly, witchcraft, or ancestors slighted as a result of broken taboos (Ashforth 2002; Ingstad 1990; Liddell *et al* 2005; Ngubane 1977; Ntloedibe-Kuswani 1999).

'Pollution' of the body is an important aspect of many African cosmo-logies. Pollutants can take two forms, environmental and ritual, both of which are understood to cause illness (Golooba-Mutebi and Tollman 2007). Dust, seen as a form of environmental pollution, is believed to cause TB, while ritual pollution is believed to be caused by a failure to observe specific conventions and rituals (Golooba-Mutebi and Tollman 2007). Ritual pollutants are often understood to originate from acts of sexual intercourse, birth or death (Ashforth 2005; Ngubane 1977; Niehaus 2001; Thomas 2008). Women are often viewed as potential sites or sources of pollution. According to traditional Zulu beliefs, men can become 'con-taminated' by debilitating pollutants if they come into contact with women who have recently given birth, miscarried or undergone terminations. Menstruating women are also considered dangerous (Ngubane 1977). Social convention in West (Oppong 1973) and East Africa (Fratkin 1996) reflects similar traditional fears of contamination from menstruating women. Contamination can result in the loss of virility, the weakening of immune systems, bad luck and misfortune. Pollution can also affect cattle; it is believed to have the effect of impeding milk production – a problem highly relevant to formerly pastoral societies. Sexual intercourse itself can be viewed as mildly polluting, becoming more so when the factors listed above come into play. Death, too, is polluting, particularly if it is unexpected (Ashforth 2005; Ngubane 1977). However, the effects of pollution can be negated if appropriate purification rituals are performed.

Given the clear links between 'pollution', women and sexual acts, it is possible to see how the symptoms of sexually-transmitted infections (STIs) may be viewed through the lens of traditional African cosmologies. This is problematic for biomedical practitioners from both a preventative and curative perspective. Traditionally, STIs have been understood to be the result of witchcraft or 'pollution' caused by violated sexual taboos – a man's intercourse with a widow, for instance, or with a woman who has recently miscarried or terminated a pregnancy. According to Zulu tradition, a cuckolded husband could punish his wife's lovers with a charm invoking STI-like symptoms (Ngubane 1977). In both Zulu and Xhosa society, the idea of the potential 'polluting effects' of women is reflected in the widespread belief that women are able to utilize their genital organs as conduits for malevolent magic. Some Zulu and Xhosa respondents have also claimed that STI-like symptoms can be caused by delayed urination and ejaculation and sex with a woman who is tense or unwilling (Meyer-Weitz *et al* 1998). In East Africa, a number of Samburu respondents have claimed that gonorrhoea can occur spontaneously if a man becomes too infatuated with an unattainable woman (Fratkin 1996). Likewise, in Liberia, some traditional healers have maintained that STIs can be transmitted through the air, through food, through contact with people recently bereaved and even through clothes (Green 1992b, 1994). Similar ideas about the transmission of STIs can be found in Ghana, Mozambique, Swaziland and Zimbabwe (Green 1992a).

Importantly, from this perspective, the sexual act itself is not necessarily the main conduit for transmission. STI's become manifest as a result of charms and the ingestation of either medicines or poisons. Even if HIV/AIDS is linked to sexual behaviour, 'safer-sex' messages focusing on condom-use are thus potentially at risk of falling on deaf ears. Ashforth (2002) argues that interrogating traditional interpretations of STIs is pointless with respect to HIV/AIDS because the diseases generally linked to AIDS in sub-Saharan Africa – tuberculosis, wasting and diarrhoea – are not traditionally linked to sex. However, attitudes to 'safer-sex' messages can nonetheless be informative. In South Africa, a 1998 survey found that respondents argued that a misplaced condom might find its way into the uterus, with fatal results. It was also claimed that condoms, being 'unnatural', could themselves provoke the recurrence of STI symptoms (Meyer-Weitz *et al* 1998). Despite Ashforth's contentions, then, the symptoms of AIDS can also potentially be understood in terms of sexual pollution. Amongst the Shiyei, Subia and Sifwe in Namibia, sexual pollution is believed to result in *kahomo*, the symptoms of which include coughing, swollen joints, diarrhoea, and wasting – all similar to symptoms experienced by AIDS sufferers (Thomas 2008). However, *kahomo* is understood to be curable if a range of stipulated purification rituals are carried out under the guidance of a traditional healer. Safer-sex messages have little resonance within this cosmology.

The 'witchcraft paradigm' offers an explanation for the poor reception of prevention strategies involving 'safer-sex' and condoms. As Christine Liddell *et al* (2005) highlight, 'it is questionable whether a single disease and a single-issue education campaign (particularly one concerning an STI) could subvert a historically grounded and responsive cosmology of illness'. According to Ashforth (2002) the 'witchcraft paradigm' allows people who have been affected by illness to derive meaning from their suffering by addressing questions such as 'why me?' and 'why now'. He argues that this worldview also allows people to make sense of a disease that affects previously fit, young, healthy and productive members of society. The fact that HIV/AIDS is an 'unjust' disease, targeting both the 'innocent and the guilty', lends weight to the idea that malevolent forces are at work.

Further social functions of the 'witchcraft paradigm'

It is not only for diagnosis and treatment that people turn to traditional healers. Witchcraft explanations also serve as socially acceptable explanations for illness. This is especially true for AIDS. The stigma with which AIDS sufferers are frequently tarred leads people to take refuge in traditional beliefs. AIDS sufferers in South Africa, particularly during in the 1990s, were often ostracized when their status became public. There were instances in which victims were lynched; in 1998 Gugu Dlamini, an early AIDS activist, was stoned to death by her community after she revealed her status on television (Iliffe 2004). In 2003, another South African AIDS activist, Lorna Mlosana, was raped and then subsequently murdered when her attacker learned of her HIV-positive status (Bhana *et al* 2004). Given that HIV/AIDS is often perceived to be self-inflicted, witchcraft explanations have the benefit of removing blame from the victim. It is for this reason that many Africans never seek confirmation of their HIV status. By the late 1990s, it was estimated that nearly 50 percent of funerals in southern Zambia were the result of AIDS, yet fewer than 3 percent of the families of the bereaved acknowledged awareness of the deceased's HIV status (Iliffe 2004). Witchcraft narratives enable victims to remain 'socially acceptable', to draw on the sympathy and support of their communities and to avoid the stigmatization of their households (Thomas 2008). Indeed, judgement by the community is one of the reasons given by respondents in areas like the Caprivi in Namibia to justify their use of traditional healers rather than biomedical practitioners (Thomas 2008).

The witchcraft paradigm can therefore protect HIV/AIDS sufferers from stigma, but there is a corresponding social downside. For every perceived victim of witchcraft, there is a perpetrator. 'Witch-hunts' continue to be problematic in many parts of sub-Saharan Africa, with many of those accused (usually elderly women) being killed by sectors of their own communities. Between 1970 and 1988, in Sukumaland, Tanzania, government figures recorded the murder of 3,072 people killed in witch-hunts. The vast majority of victims – over 80 percent – were women between the ages of 50 and 60 (Miguel 2004). In May 2008 in Kenya, eight women and three men, the majority aged between 70 and 90, were burnt to death by a mob convinced that they were witches (Federici 2008). Thousands of elderly women in Ghana have banded together in 'witch camps' in order to protect themselves from accusations of witchcraft and sorcery (UN 2006b). The elderly are frequently targeted because witches are believed to be motivated by jealousy, and elderly women, especially widows, are viewed as being envious of those younger than them and are thus obvious targets. Another purported signifier is having red eyes and elderly women, having spent decades indoors tending poorly-ventilated fires, often suffer from this condition (Adinkrah 2004). Ghana has become notorious for its persecution of witches, with a number of high profile 'witch-hunts' placing traditional belief systems under the spotlight. In 1997, there was a severe outbreak of cerebrospinal meningitis in the northern region of the country that resulted in over 500 deaths (Adinkrah 2004). Suspicions of witchcraft led to a number of elderly women being beaten and stoned to death. These women, usually widows, have no financial resources and are wholly dependent on family members for subsistence. Given the paucity of social welfare programmes in Ghana, elderly women expelled from their communities and forced to flee to 'witch-camps' become extremely vulnerable (Adinkrah 2004). However, it is not only the elderly who are at risk. In West Africa, children are frequently accused of witchcraft, which can result in physical abuse and ostracism (Stobart 2006). It is possible to see a similar pattern in central and southern Africa. In Kinshasa in the DRC, there are estimated to be approximately 100,000 street children. Almost half of these are said to have been abandoned following accusations of witchcraft (Cahn 2006). In Angola, the UN has reported instances of children as young as five being sexually abused, stoned, hanged and drowned as witches (cited in Home Office 2005).

The role of traditional healers

The fact that societies that view disease through the prism of the 'witchcraft paradigm' are vulnerable to the misdiagnosis of HIV/AIDS means that the role of traditional healers, as cornerstones within the cosmology, must be considered crucial to overcoming the potential dangers of this worldview. This is a challenge acknowledged by the WHO (2002), UNAIDS (2000b) and the World Bank (2004). However, despite optimistic documents like that commemorating five years of the World Bank's (2004) Indigenous Knowledge Programme, which celebrates increasing cooperation between traditional healers and biomedicine, co-opting this sector to help fight HIV/AIDS has proven difficult. For policymakers working to exploit the influence and standing of traditional healers in the community, there is a complex challenge involved in bringing what many people would perceive to be superstition and 'snake oil' remedies within a largely informal sector, into the rigid structures of the formal healthcare sector. In order to fight HIV/AIDS and improve general access to healthcare, a number of African countries have attempted to legislate and regulate traditional healers and practitioners of traditional medicine (WHO 2002).

African traditional healers can be generally classified as either diviners or herbalists, the former engaging with supernatural matters and the latter being responsible for the production of traditional remedies. However, the dedicated herbalist, who might be comparable to a 'western-style' pharmacist, is somewhat rare and, as a result, the public does not readily distinguish between diviners and herbalists (Ashforth 2005). Most of the time, the line between the two is thin. For instance, amongst the Batswana a healer who is incapable of acting as a diviner is perceived to be 'incomplete' (Ntloedibe-Kuswani 1999). Few herbalists actively disassociate their treatments from the 'witchcraft paradigm'. Many herbalists in East Africa ascribe 'magical powers' to their cures (Iliffe 1998). In West Africa, amongst the Hausa in Nigeria, the term 'traditional healer' incorporates magician-healers (*boka*) and herbalists (*mai magani*), as well as barber-surgeons (*wanzami*), bonesetters (*mad'ori*) and Koranic scholar-healers – all of whom claim to draw much of their healing power from supernatural forces (Stock 1981).

The extent to which the supernatural lies at the heart of the traditional healers' oeuvre is evident from attempts made to formalize the training and registration of 'legitimate' traditional healers. As outlined in Chapter 4, when it came to combating HIV/AIDS the Mbeki administration in South Africa was anxious to explore the idea of an 'African solution to an African problem'. Seeking an alternative strategy for the treatment of HIV/AIDS, the South African government became an enthusiastic supporter of the potential role of traditional medicine. However, when the government set forth its Traditional Health Practitioners Bill in 2003, it had to confront the complexities of prescribing the qualifications necessary to become a traditional healer. Within Zulu tradition, anyone wishing to qualify as a herbalist (*inyanga*) had to be apprenticed to an established practitioner for at least a year, but the traditional qualifications for becoming a diviner (*isangoma*) are less quantifiable from a bureaucratic perspective. Diviners were 'chosen' by the ancestors and, while novices may have trained with an established *isangoma*, much of their knowledge was 'revealed' to them in dreams or visions (Ashforth 2005; Ngubane 1977). Similar problems are evident in Nigeria where herbal remedies tended to be revealed to Hausa practitioners through dreams (Stock 1981). Any state attempt to formalize and regulate the sector through the development of 'best practice' is thus fraught with difficulty. Where the South African Traditional Health Practitioners Bill attempted to clarify the state position on the qualifications necessary to operate as a licensed traditional practitioner, it was vague to the point of meaninglessness:

> The Minister may, on the recommendation of the council, prescribe qualifications obtained by virtue of examinations conducted by an accredited institution, educational authority or other examining authority in the Republic, which, held singly or conjointly with any other qualification shall entitle any holder thereof to registration in terms of this Act if he or she has, before or in connection with or after the acquisition of the qualification in question, complied with such conditions or requirements as may be prescribed (South African Government 2003).

Defining what constitutes an 'authentic' healer is thus hugely problematic. As a compromise, the South African state and others including

Ghana and Nigeria have attempted to 'professionalize' the sector. In Ghana, the Kwame Nkrumah University of Science and Technology offers a Bachelor's Degree in Herbal Medicine. The Zambia Institute for Natural Medicine and Research (WHO 2009f) offers a Doctor of Naturopathic Medicine qualification. Burkina Faso, Ghana, Mali, Senegal, Uganda and Tanzania also offer institutionalized training programmes for traditional health practitioners. However, professionalization measures, by their very nature, negate much within African traditional medicine that is inherently unquantifiable.

That so much of what qualifies a person to be a traditional healer is so esoteric makes it difficult to separate authentic healers from charlatans. For instance, the controversial South African *uBhejane* (rhino) herbal 'cure' was 'revealed' in a dream to Zeblon Gwala, formerly a truck driver, by his late grandfather, who had been a traditional healer (TAC 2008). Gwala's newspaper advertisements claimed that his concoction 'increases your CD4 count and reduces the viral load until it disappears' (ASA 2008). A Medical University study found the herbal mixture to have no effect on HIV (Doctors for Life 2006). Problematically, Gwala's patients were told that they could not take ARVs and *uBhejane* in conjunction with one another (TAC 2008).

From a biomedical perspective, efforts to identify 'charlatans' are not necessarily sufficient where the diagnosis and treatment of HIV/AIDS is concerned. The major concern lies with the cosmology itself. According to the 'witchcraft paradigm' there are, arguably, no incurable diseases like HIV/AIDS because, if the disease is caused by some form of 'sorcery', then it can be combated accordingly. Controversially, the South African Act provides healers with the opportunity to make diagnoses and to offer 'cures' incorporating elements of sorcery, so long as they are officially registered as traditional practitioners. The Act merely makes it illegal for unregistered healers to make similar claims:

(i) diagnoses, treats or offers to treat, or prescribes treatment or any cure for, cancer, HIV and AIDS or any other prescribed terminal disease;

(ii) holds himself or herself out to be able to treat or cure cancer, HIV and AIDS or any other prescribed terminal disease or to prescribe treatment therefore; or

(iii) holds out that any article, compound, traditional medicine or apparatus is or may be of value for the alleviation, curing or treatment of cancer, HIV and AIDS or any other prescribed terminal disease (South African Government 2003).

The *uBhejane* case is only one amongst many. Advertisements for HIV/ AIDS 'cures' plaster the walls of innumerable African cities and have been widely marketed in newspapers (Flint 2009j; Nattrass 2008; Orubuloye and Oguntimehin 1999).

Efficacy of traditional medicine

Even if the 'witchcraft' or sorcery element is removed and traditional health practitioners are viewed instead as guardians of indigenous knowledge systems, there is to date no clinical evidence that suggests that any traditional African remedies are effective against HIV/AIDS in the long term. Traditional healers advertising a cure for HIV/AIDS are not necessarily consciously setting out to defraud patients; neither would they view themselves as charlatans. Claims made for a cure are frequently tied to a traditional view of disease that, for the vast majority of traditional healers and their patients, suggests that an absence of symptoms equates to a cure (Wreford 2005). Clearly, such a position is deeply problematic where HIV/AIDS is concerned. By treating opportunistic infections and boosting appetites, many traditional healers can achieve short-term success, thereby 'healing' patients. Problematically, patients who believe themselves to be 'cured' of HIV are unlikely to take ARVs and engage in 'safer-sex' practices.

From the above, it is evident that regulating or professionalizing a sector that has at its heart elements of the supernatural is problematic for policymakers. In some instances, traditional medicines have proved successful in the treatment of diseases such as malaria, sickle cell-disease and hypertension. Traditional fever remedies derived from willow (*Salix alba*), cinchona (*Cinchona succirubra*), and quin hao (*Artemisia annua*) have proved effective as anti-inflammatory agents (Okpako 1999). However, given that HIV/AIDS is a relatively new disease, there is little to suggest that traditional medicine would be effective in combating it – it is not a traditional African ailment and therefore there is no reason to presuppose a time-honoured response. The determination by some African states to find an 'African solution' has resulted in a scramble to find a traditional cure. As stated, despite a number of high-profile contenders, there is no scientific evidence to suggest that any traditional African remedies are capable of offering successful treatment. ARVs remain the only proven regimen for the disease (Pekala 2007). The truth is that traditional remedies can be toxic, and sometimes fatally so. A 2002 study in *Human & Experimental Toxicology* reports that across Africa traditional medicine is a major cause of hospitalization (Tagwireyi *et al* 2002). An epidemiological study of acute poisoning admissions to the Ga-Rankuwa Hospital in Pretoria between 1981 and 1985 revealed that, of the fatalities considered, the majority (51.7 percent) of deaths were caused by the consumption of traditional medicine (Joubert 1990). Estimates suggest that in South Africa alone traditional medicine results in thousands of deaths every year (Popat *et al* 2001). It is difficult to ascertain a more accurate figure because many of those who rely on traditional medicines live in rural areas and are without access to allopathic care; death by poisoning is often not recorded as such (Popat *et al* 2001).

It is not unusual for traditional medicines to contain natural toxins, including extracts of *Euphorbia* (wartweed), *Solanum* (nightshade), *Datura* (Jamestown weed) and *Ricinis communis* (castorbean) as well as cantharides (Spanish Fly) (Tagwireyi *et al* 2002). *Callilepis laureola* (ox-eye daisy) is a herb common to Zulu remedies. Usually drunk as a tea, it is used to treat upset stomachs and menstrual cramps, and eradicate tape worm, cure impotence and improve fertility. It is also used in deliveries by traditional birth attendants and is said to ward off malevolent spirits (Popat *et al* 2001). *Callilepis laureola* has been found to be extremely toxic and may be the cause of an estimated 1,500 deaths per year (Popat *et al* 2001). Critically, the scope for poisoning is aggravated substantially by the fact that there are no prescribed dosages, and healers are frequently vague when prescribing quantities for ingestion. This is especially problematic with respect to young children, whose bodies are often unable to cope with adult dosages. Many herbal toxins are difficult to screen for and patients are often unaware of what they have consumed (Stewart *et al* 1999). Problematic, too, is that two herbs common to traditional remedies across southern Africa appear to interfere with the efficacy and metabolism of some ARVs (Van den Bout-van den Beukel *et al* 2006). *Hypoxis* (African Potato) is used to treat urinary infections, heart weakness, tumours, nervous disorders, and immune-related illnesses, including HIV/AIDS. *Sutherlandia* (Cancer Bush) is used to treat cancers, tuberculosis, diabetes, influenza, depression and HIV/AIDS. Given that departments of health in Angola, Botswana, Democratic Republic of Congo, Lesotho, Malawi, Mauritius, Mozambique, Namibia, Seychelles, South Africa, Swaziland, Tanzania, Zambia, and Zimbabwe have endorsed these two herbs as appropriate to the treatment of HIV/AIDS, it is imperative that the efficacy of these treatments be established (Mills *et al* 2005).

Enemas are a widespread traditional treatment for many health problems, including psychosis, headaches, gonorrhoea and constipation. In the past, it was common for Swazi babies to receive up to 50 enemas a year (Dunn *et al* 1991; Kale 1995); they remain a frequently-prescribed treatment for diarrhoea (Seidal 2005). Ingredients used in enemas commonly include non-herbal toxins like metal salts or ores: arsenic, copper sulphate and potassium dichromate (Steenkamp *et al* 2002; Steenkamp 2002). In addition, despite certain preconceptions, not all 'traditional remedies' have historical pedigrees. They may be neither uniformly 'natural' nor organic. Traditional practitioners, particularly in urban areas, have proved willing to experiment with 'modern' ingredients. Potassium permanganate, used in electroplating, tanning, cement manufacture and photographic processing, is referred to in Xhosa as a 'cure for all ills' (Dunn *et al* 1991). In South Africa, thinners, turpentine, chloroxylenol antiseptic, ginger, pepper, soap, vinegar and caustics have all been found to be components in enemas administered by traditional healers.

To overcome questions pertaining to the value of traditional medicines, the South African government moved to have such remedies clinically tested for 'efficacy, safety and quality ... with a view to incorporating their use in the healthcare system' (South African Government 1996a). In 1997, the Medical Research Council, with funding of R4.5 million from the Ministry of Health, created a Traditional Medicines Research Unit (Mills 2006). The *uBhejane* herbal 'cure' for HIV/AIDS mentioned above was a high profile casualty of demands for western-style testing. *UBhejane* was trialled by the Medical University in South Africa in 2005. Despite being advocated beforehand by then South African health minister Tshabalala-Msimang, Peggy Nkonyeni, the KwaZulu-Natal Province Health MEC (member of the executive council), and the mayor of eThekwini (which incorporates the major urban centre of Durban), the Medical University found the herbal mixture to have no effect in the treatment of HIV/AIDS. Tshabalala-Msimang (2007), famous for her support of alternative therapies for HIV/AIDS (Chapter 4), spoke out against perceived attempts by the biomedical establishment to prevent, through testing protocols, the 'mainstreaming of African traditional medicine'. She argued that proven efficacy was unnecessary and that 'we cannot use Western models of protocols for research and development. We should guard against getting bogged down with clinical trials' (*Mail and Guardian* 24/02/2008).

As part of its programme of engagement with indigenous knowledge systems, the South African Medical Research Council conducted toxicity tests on a number of herbs and herbal combinations. *Sutherlandia* (Seier *et al* 2002) and LEAF, a mixture of *Hypoxis* (African potato), milk thistle, Beta-sitosterol/plant sterols and *Spirulina* (Mdhluli *et al* 2004) have been shown to be non-toxic. However, evidence of their supposed efficacy in managing HIV/AIDS remains largely anecdotal. Consequently, despite concerted attempts to demonstrate the value of traditional alternatives to ARV treatment, there is little to no evidence to suggest that these remedies have any noticeable effect on combating HIV/AIDS. In fact, at best, they appear to do no harm. In African countries, governmental support for traditional remedies for HIV/AIDS simply creates confusion in the minds of those seeking effective treatment (Chapter 4).

Bringing traditional healers and traditional medicine on side

Continuing support for traditional healers has forced governments and international donor agencies to recognize the potential of the former to assist with HIV/AIDS diagnosis and treatment. A number of African countries have legislated to recognize the role played by traditional practitioners in providing healthcare. Ghana and Nigeria have an inclusive approach to traditional medicine. Both countries have a national policy on the subject and a unit or department within the ministry of health responsible for overseeing the sector (WHO 2002). Nigeria has even integrated traditional medicine into its official healthcare system. Ghana, meanwhile, has worked to ensure that the majority of its 45,000 traditional healers are recognized and licensed with the Ghana Federation of Traditional Medicine Practitioners' Association, and that the safety of traditional remedies is overseen (Romero-Daza 2002). Across the continent, there is a growing trend towards collaborative projects between traditional healers and biomedical practitioners.

However, 'AIDS entrepreneurship' and a worldview that is seemingly at odds with the accepted tenets of Western medicine has resulted in scepticism concerning the value of traditional healers in attempting to stem the tide of HIV/AIDS. The South Africa-based group Doctors for Life, an NGO consisting of local and international biomedical practitioners, has been especially vocal in articulating such doubts, demanding appropriate science-based testing for all traditional medicine. Spokesman Dr Moses Thindisa has argued that:

> We do accept the fact that they have been here from time immemorial and that they won't disappear. But we would like their medications to be tested in laboratories before being given to the people. But

unfortunately for now their medication remains untested. At some point you find that some people get sick and have to be treated in hospitals after taking untested medications (cited in Ngcobo 2007).

An insistence on scientific rigour and clinical testing is problematic with respect to bringing the two medical communities together, yet biomedical campaigners insist that this is essential if traditional remedies are to be brought into the mainstream. Conversely, Joanne Wreford (2008a, 2008b), an anthropologist and traditional healer based at the University of Cape Town, argues that such attitudes are unnecessarily divisive and that biomedical practitioners need come to view traditional healers as allies rather than rivals. Wreford (2008a) maintains that 'if the communication that does take place insists on scientific supremacy and refuses reciprocity, the effort is likely to disappoint' and that 'it is vital ... that western trained medical personnel start to make serious, and respectful efforts to connect intellectually with the ideas that underline traditional practice'. Wreford infers that, by refusing to engage with traditional healers other than on their own terms, biomedical practitioners risk alienating potential collaborators.

Where traditional healers and biomedical practitioners have been brought together, the results have sometimes been encouraging. In Uganda, under the auspices of the Traditional and Modern Health Practitioners Together against AIDS and Other Diseases (THETA) initiative, established in 1992, a small group of traditional healers completed a 15-month course on HIV/AIDS and was then asked to apply this training to their practices. Of those who participated on the course, which ran from 1997 to 1998, 97 percent subsequently referred patients suspected of having HIV/AIDS to biomedical practitioners (UNAIDS 2000b). A similar collaboration in Tanzania dubbed the Tanga AIDS Working Group (TAWG), also founded in 1992, saw a dramatic increase in referrals and vastly improved condoms sales in areas where the group was active (Prakash 2005; UNAIDS 2000b). These projects, together with comparable collaborations in Botswana, Malawi, Mozambique, South Africa and Zambia demonstrate the potential for traditional healers and biomedical practitioners to cooperate in a meaningful manner. However, most such collaborations are not 'meetings of minds'. Rather, they are establishment attempts to impose a more biomedical paradigm on traditional healers. As Wreford (2005) has argued, there is very little evidence of true exchange. In essence, for collaborations to succeed, traditional healers need to acknowledge the primacy of western medicine. This suggests that a true reconciliation between the two schools is impossible and that, at best, traditional medicine can be accommodated only in a relatively nominal manner.

Conclusion

The issue of witchcraft has long been a sensitive subject with respect to Africa. In English, and other European languages, it is difficult to disengage 'witchcraft' from connotations of 'backwardness', 'superstition' and 'irrationality'. Terms such as 'witch-doctor' have become decidedly politically incorrect. Accordingly, there has been a temptation to avoid engaging with the subject. Cultural relativity is vital, given the atrocities of the colonial era, especially so with respect to sub-Saharan Africa. Certain donors and development agencies like the WHO (2002) and the World Bank (2004), have tended to ignore certain 'culturally sensitive' issues linked to the treatment of disease in Africa. Instead, we have seen the creation of 'traditional medicine strategies' (WHO) and the 'Indigenous Knowledge for Development Programme' (World Bank) which, regardless of their considerable merit in other areas, conveniently bypass any real engagement with underlying cosmologies and value-systems.

The fact that up to 80 percent of people living in Africa consult traditional healers is a clear indication of the importance and influence of the latter in determining the treatment of many illnesses, including HIV/AIDS. A desire to reconcile traditional healers and biomedical practitioners is thus an obvious step within HIV/AIDS governance. There are, however, a number of problems associated with this approach, the most important of which pertains to 'indigenous representations of disease'. A belief system that understands illness, disease and death to be linked to witchcraft and malicious intent by malevolent individuals is deeply problematic for those preaching a message of behaviour change or even, simply, risk aversion (Chapters 6 and 7). While concepts such as 'sexual pollution' are compatible with many African cosmologies, and HIV/AIDS could be 'framed' in such a manner, the simple fact remains that, in Africa, sexually-transmitted diseases are often viewed through the prism of a 'witchcraft paradigm'. The notion that sorcery is perceived to be specific to the intended victim makes the idea of a sexually-transmitted pandemic hard to conceptualize. This means that the urgency of prevention messages often fails to convince intended audiences. It has been argued that the 'witchcraft paradigm' serves a number of positive functions. It prevents the stigmatization of those suffering from HIV/AIDS and, by imposing order on seemingly random events, answers the questions 'why me?'

and 'why now?'. However, as has been demonstrated, there is another side to this coin: across the continent, in countries including Angola, DRC, Ghana, Kenya, South Africa and Tanzania, those perceived to be responsible for exercising witchcraft, usually elderly women, have been persecuted by their communities and even killed.

Assessing traditional medicines and traditional healers in relation to the treatment and management of HIV/AIDS gives rise to a number of uncomfortable problems. Despite the best efforts of the South African government to find clinical evidence for the efficacy of traditional medicines in treating HIV/AIDS, there are no quantifiable data to suggest that any of these remedies are in any way useful. At best, these medicines may be non-toxic. The past determination of elements within the South African Ministry of Health to afford traditional medicine a status that it does not warrant is irresponsible in the extreme. In the midst of a pandemic of unprecedented proportions, former Health Minister Tshabala-Msimang's comments that traditional medicines should be exempt from the rigours of clinical testing, and her support for remedies revealed to would-be pharmacists *via* 'conversations' with deceased relatives (the *uBhejane* example) make for uncomfortable reading. In many instances, healers have demonstrated considerable entrepreneurial skill in marketing their cures and, more worryingly, in persuading those infected with HIV to forgo ARV treatment.

Any attempt to regulate the sub-Saharan traditional medicine sector is fraught with difficulty. After all, 'witch-doctors' are 'selected' by ancestors to fulfil their calling, rather than trained in the biomedical sense. While apprenticeships are frequently served, especially by dedicated herbalists, the majority of practitioners' remedies have supernatural rather than scientific origins. Such issues make distinguishing between genuine traditional healers and charlatans extremely difficult and formal accreditation in any meaningful sense almost impossible. This distinction is made more difficult by virtue of the fact that many traditional healers who claim to be able to cure HIV/AIDS are neither fraudsters nor 'quacks'; they themselves genuinely believe in their ability. The nature of HIV/AIDS augments this. For the majority of traditional practitioners, the absence of symptoms equates to evidence of a cure and, by virtue of this fact, the successful treatment of opportunistic infections can be claimed, in good faith, to be effective treatment for HIV/AIDS.

If regulation of the sector is beset with potential policy landmines, then so too are attempts at collaboration between traditional and biomedical practitioners. 'Successful' examples all involve the co-option and 'education' of traditional healers. Success (in terms of integration within the biomedical sphere) is measured by an increased flow of people within a particular community to clinics for testing, and increased levels of ARV- and condom-usage. However, it is difficult to perceive a two-way flow of ideas within this model of 'collaboration'. Where HIV/AIDS is concerned, I have been unable to locate examples of biomedical practitioners adopting indigenous African interpretations of disease; neither have I found instances of biomedical shifts from positions of scientific best practice to ones governed by one or more aspects of the 'witchcraft paradigm'. Existing traditional/biomedical cooperation is, in essence, missionary work, and to pretend otherwise is simply to pay lip service to notions of cultural relativity and concerns regarding cultural insensitivity and racism. The fact remains that the only proven method for managing HIV/AIDS is through the administration of ARVs and the promulgation of sound prevention strategies. The 'witchcraft paradigm', whilst coherent, rational and entrenched, is potentially dangerous with respect to both treatment programmes and prevention efforts. Cultural-sensitivity squeamishness should not result in lives being lost. Across Africa, there is potential for traditional healers to form a critical aspect of the wider biomedical healthcare superstructure. At the same time, pretending that traditional medicine is somehow equivalent to allopathic treatments at best encourages confusion and at worst results in further increases in infection and, ultimately, mortality rates.

6
The International Response: Multilateral and Unilateral Approaches

The international community was slow to respond to HIV/AIDS in sub-Saharan Africa. For much of the 1980s and 1990s, funding remained limited. However, pressure to respond to the crisis led to the formation of three key donor programmes:

- The World Bank's Multi-Country HIV/AIDS Program for Africa (MAP), established in 2001,
- The Global Fund to Fight AIDS, Tuberculosis and Malaria (henceforth 'Global Fund'), operational since 2002,
- The US President's Emergency Plan for AIDS Relief (PEPFAR), authorized in 2003.

Of the three programmes, MAP and the Global Fund are multilateral initiatives, while PEPFAR is assiduously unilateral in its approach. The existence of three competing agencies, similar in focus and remit, and operating in the same theatre, has proved controversial; critics have pointed to overlapping constituencies, duplication and a lack of coordination. This chapter evaluates these contrasting international init-iatives and their impact in shaping governance and the nature of treatment and prevention programmes in sub-Saharan Africa. In contrast to the post-Washington Consensus trend for project 'ownership', as implicit in MAP and Global Fund ventures, PEPFAR adopted an unashamedly 'hands-on' approach to project management in sub-Saharan Africa. Given the sensitivity on the part of many African elites to suggestions of neo-imperialism, PEPFAR was, and remains, tantamount to a 'throwback' to a previous era of development politics. PEPFAR represents itself as a proudly American initiative and a moral force for good in the world. It is 'old-fashioned' in other respects; it was launched in 2003 from a clear moral platform that prioritized the conservative Christian values of abstinence and fidelity over more 'democratic', less judgemental approaches to HIV/AIDS involving 'safer sex' messages. At the same time, in terms of funding, the monies made available to PEPFAR, $15 billion at its launch in 2003 and $48 billion at its re-authorization in 2008, have been unprecedented. The net result is that the 'largest commitment ever by a single nation toward an international health initiative' (PEPFAR 2009a) has also resurrected old debates involving North-South inequalities and the imposition of 'missionary values'.

PEPFAR, MAP and the Global Fund

In January 2003, in his State of the Union address, President Bush announced the introduction of PEPFAR, calling on Congress to approve funding of $15 billion to combat HIV/AIDS, malaria and tuberculosis in Africa and the Caribbean. The United States Leadership against HIV/AIDS, Tuberculosis and Malaria Act of 2003, which established PEPFAR, was duly passed by Congress in May of that year and the first funds became available in January 2004. The plan was subsequently reauthorized in July 2008, this time with a budget of $48 billion to be spread over five years. The HIV/AIDS funding authorized in 2003, of which 80 percent was aimed at care and treatment, were allocated as follows (US Government 2003a):

(1) 55 percent of such amounts for treatment of individuals with HIV/AIDS;
(2) 15 percent of such amounts for palliative care of individuals with HIV/AIDS;
(3) 20 percent of such amounts for HIV/AIDS prevention … of which such amount at least 33 percent should be expended for abstinence until-marriage programs; and
(4) 10 percent of such amounts for orphans and vulnerable children.

The 2008 reauthorization, less prescriptive than its predecessor, particularly with respect to prevention programmes, had a similarly treatment-based focus. The Act places an emphasis on treatment, with more than half of monies to be spent on the following five areas:

(1) antiretroviral treatment for HIV/AIDS;
(2) clinical monitoring of HIV-seropositive people not in need of antiretroviral treatment;
(3) care for associated opportunistic infections;

(4) nutrition and food support for people living with HIV/AIDS; and

(5) other essential HIV/AIDS-related medical care for people living with HIV/AIDS.

The 2008 project targeted 15 'focus' countries in Africa, Asia and the Caribbean, namely Botswana, Cote d'Ivoire, Ethiopia, Guyana, Haiti, Kenya, Mozambique, Namibia, Nigeria, Rwanda, South Africa, Tanzania, Uganda, Vietnam and Zambia. These countries were targeted because of their high levels of prevalence and limited resources. However, PEPFAR funds to combat HIV/AIDS have also been made available to other 'non-focus' developing countries including India (although relations between India and the US with regard to HIV/AIDS are complex – Chapter 8).

PEPFAR has come under criticism for being aggressively unilateral in its approach to rolling out its programme, and questions have been raised as to the necessity of maintaining three separate initiatives operating within the same field, which has inevitably given rise to problems relating to duplication and a lack of co-ordination. In many respects the debate is one centred on efficiency. Whilst PEPFAR is nominally top-down in approach and ideologically motivated, its apologists claim that the programme holds a number of advantages over the Global Fund and MAP: security of funding, relatively prompt decision-making, clear-cut priorities, transparent purchasing and distribution systems, and vigorous oversight.

Both MAP and the Global Fund predate PEPFAR. MAP, an initiative of the World Bank and the smallest of the three initiatives in terms of both scope and funding, was established in 2001. Between the financial years 2001 and 2006, the World Bank committed $1.286 billion to combating HIV/AIDS in Africa (Görgens-Albino *et al* 2007). MAP was designed to be more flexible than traditional World Bank projects, and more responsive to changing circumstances (Görgens-Albino *et al* 2007). MAP offers grants, loans or credits, often at zero interest, to countries that meet World Bank eligibility criteria for funding. Recipient states must demonstrate both a willingness to work with civil society and stakeholder groups and a capacity to coordinate between these interest groups. The World Bank has been at pains to emphasize the speed with which MAP funds can be rolled out. In the past, project-based support required, on average, 18 months before funds became available. Through MAP, the Bank was able to cut this waiting period by half (Görgens-Albino *et al* 2007).

Established in 2002, the Global Fund is a public-private partnership combining funding from approximately 50 countries (Global Fund 2007) with monies raised by private initiatives including (PRODUCT) RED, fronted by the rock group U2's lead singer, Bono. The initiative encourages businesses to brand products with the RED logo, the profits of which are then channelled to the Global Fund. Brand names that have signed up to the venture include American Express, Apple, Converse, GAP, Microsoft and Starbucks. The tying of consumerism to philanthropy is difficult to reconcile for many people but given that, as of April 2010, RED had raised $140 million for the Global Fund (RED 2010), it may sometimes be a case of the end justifying the means. The Global Fund was initially administered through the World Health Organization (WHO) but became an autonomous administrative organization in 2009. The body is active in 140 countries and has generated $19.3 billion in funding since its establishment (Global Fund 2010). Countries wishing to secure grants from the Global Fund must establish Country Coordinating Mechanisms (CCMs) that are responsible for both negotiating levels of funding and the monitoring and management of approved monies. Once approved, funds are distributed through the Principal Recipient (PR), usually a government department with an independent Local Fund Agent (LFA) appointed to every PR in order to ensure correct oversight.

One of the criticisms levelled at PEPFAR is that, compared to the other two initiatives, it adopts a vigorous top-down approach, something that is at odds with current donor practices encouraging 'ownership' of projects. PEPFAR also tends to work with partner organizations rather than through specific government channels. Governments can apply for PEPFAR funding but have to claim and account for monies in the same way as any NGO partner organization. PEPFAR initiatives are overseen by US federal employees, and recipient country governments are only involved peripherally (Oomman *et al* 2007). PEPFAR's unilateral approach is in stark contrast to the other two programmes, which allow for a far greater degree of recipient country ownership. Where the Global Fund is concerned, recipient governments play an important role in planning and overseeing the distribution of funds via its Country Coordinating Mechanism. The World Bank's MAP initiative involves recipient governments to an even greater degree, designing and distributing funds in conjunction with World Bank staff (Oomman *et al* 2007). The South African government in particular has voiced its discomfort regarding PEPFAR's sidelining of the state. In 2006, then South African Health Minister Tshabalala-Msimang complained about a lack of consultation, expressing the government's surprise that South Africa had even been nominated as a PEPFAR focus country three years previously. It was claimed that no consultation between the two governments had taken place (*Mail and*

Guardian 12/06/2006). In order to rectify what she perceived as PEPFAR 'getting off on the wrong foot' in South Africa, Tshabalala-Msimang argued for greater coordination of external funding 'through government structures' (cited in *Mail and Guardian* 12/06/2006). However, by sidelining governments and remaining 'hands-on', it can be argued that PEPFAR has avoided the type of governance problems which have beset the Global Fund in countries including Chad, Kenya, Myanmar, Nigeria, Uganda, Ukraine and Zimbabwe.

PEPFAR has been very successful in Uganda, which has a reputation as a 'donor darling' and as an HIV/AIDS success story (Chapter 7). Yet, from a Global Fund perspective, Uganda's image is very different. In 2005, Uganda had its Global Fund grants suspended due to accounting 'irregularities'. The Fund auditors, PricewaterhouseCoopers, discovered evidence of 'serious mismanagement' of funds by elements within Uganda's Project Management Unit, overseen by the Ugandan Ministry of Health. In a press release, the Global Fund (2005) detailed that:

> PriceWaterhouseCoopers and the Global Fund Secretariat have serious concerns about inadequate monitoring and accounting of grant expenditures by the PMU and by some (not all) sub-recipients. In accounting documentation provided ... some expenses were inappropriate, unexplained or improperly documented. In addition, the criteria set out for the vetting of sub-recipients were not followed completely. For example, some entities that did not provide evidence of their legal status were awarded grants.

The Local Fund Agent, the Global Fund's designated representative, decided not to pursue a wider investigation into corruption or fraud on the part of members of the Project Management Unit, stating that there was 'no evidence of corruption or fraud'. There was, however, 'evidence of inappropriate expenditure and improper accounting' (Global Fund 2005). It was only after the Ugandan Ministry of Finance agreed to put additional oversight structures in place that funding was resumed. The Global Fund also ran into problems in Zimbabwe where, in 2007, in the midst of economic collapse and with little access to foreign exchange reserves, the Zimbabwean Reserve Bank 'quarantined' $12.3 million of Global Fund monies, refusing access to these funds for nearly a year (Global Fund 2008). Such examples bring the matter of 'good governance' sharply into focus. The fact that PEPFAR has elected to sidestep the matter completely by retaining direct control can be viewed as 'imperialistic' and indicative of the hierarchical imbalances in North-South relations. Nonetheless, taking the above examples into account, this direct approach does appear to have paid dividends.

Be this as it may, American unilateralism in the field of HIV/AIDS has engendered concern. Questions have been raised as to the need for three separate donor programmes operating in the same region. There is also a fear that multiple agencies might undermine or impede one another's operations. Furthermore, the costs incurred as a result of maintaining three bureaucratic structures might be better spent on treatment and prevention. Parallel structures, replication and competing agendas are all potentially wasteful. In terms of governance, a lack of coordination between the three initiatives has led to multiple coordination structures in the majority of recipient countries. A southern African study, conducted by Johanna Hanefield (2009) and linked to the Global HIV/AIDS Initiatives' Network, suggests that coordination between the three bodies is indeed problematic. Evidence from Zambia and South Africa indicates that, despite concerted attempts to improve coordination at the national level by the relevant governments and the agencies themselves, communication between the disparate actors remains inconsistent. The lack of coordination is exacerbated yet further at the sub-national level (Hanefeld 2009). A similar picture emerges elsewhere – in Mozambique, for instance – providing a snapshot of the difficulties inherent in coordinating and reconciling policymaking emanating from three very different funding templates. There are also indications that competition between PEPFAR, the Global Fund and MAP has resulted in skewed data sets and a distorted impression of the efficacy of the respective programmes. Anecdotal evidence from Uganda seems to suggests that a great deal of 'double counting' takes place in the areas where all three are active (Oomman *et al* 2008). In effect, a single, multilateral agency, funded by the international community would have more legitimacy and less ideological 'baggage' than, say, PEPFAR operating independently. However, evidence suggests the need for far tighter oversight than that currently offered by the Global Fund model – something that would be difficult to achieve within the current multilateral framework of the latter.

Quantifying the efficacy of PEPFAR

While a comprehensive appreciation of the impact of PEPFAR remains some years off, some indication of its success or otherwise as it currently stands would go some way toward easing concerns as to the governance of AIDS-focused funding. In addition to its unapologetically unilateral approach in the face of the more multilateral Global Fund and MAP, its prevention strategies have drawn a great deal of ire due to the importance it has attached to abstinence – a strategy that critics argue is likely to, at best, be ineffective and, at worst, actually put lives at risk. Whilst nominally centred on the ubiquitous 'ABC' (Abstain, Be faithful, use Condoms) approach, the initiative has been criticized as being 'Anything But Condoms' in its perspective. Further criticism has been levelled at PEPFAR's tendency to privilege faith-based organizations. As a result, the reauthorization of PEPFAR in 2008 was less prescriptive than the legislation approved in 2003. This, together with the election of Democrat Barack Obama in the 2008 US Presidential elections also served to ameliorate many critics' fears, with the then Presidential candidate declaring in 2008 that HIV/AIDS prevention strategies would, under his leadership, be governed by 'best practice, not ideology' (cited in Walker 2009). Likewise, Obama's nomination of the less 'ideologically-minded' Dr Eric Goosby as US Global AIDS Coordinator in early 2009 was a further indication that PEPFAR's moral compass was starting to shift.

The abstinence approach favoured by George W Bush has been one of risk elimination rather than risk reduction. As the President famously remarked, abstinence is 'the only 100 percent effective means of preventing pregnancy, HIV, and sexually-transmitted infections' (Bush 2004). Proponents argue that in poorer countries, where people are living on less than $1 per day, condoms are likely to be difficult to access and not always readily available (Boler and Ingham 2007). To this end, the first authorization of PEPFAR in 2003 dictated that a third of all funds dedicated to prevention be spent on abstinence-only programmes (US Government 2003a).

That new infections continue to outpace the generation of effective treatments means that risk education is paramount. However, despite changes in PEPFAR's mandate since its reauthorization, critics argue that its narrow worldview continues to compromise the efficacy of risk education (Morgan 2009). In particular, there is very limited evidence to suggest that abstinence programmes are successful in delaying sexual debut, and even less evidence to suggest that such programmes have been effective in sub-Saharan Africa (Kaiser Family Foundation 2005a; Trenholm *et al* 2007; Willcox 2008). While abstinence-education programmes are no longer a compulsory element of prevention strategies undertaken by PEPFAR partner organizations, the rules governing PEPFAR funding continue to demand that any 'opt-outs' be justified.

Evidence suggests that abstinence programmes tend to send out mixed messages regarding condom usage. Research in South Africa's Eastern Cape Province indicates that high school students are confused as to the reliability and efficacy of condoms as protection against HIV/AIDS (Flint 2009f, 2009g, 2009h). Participants in an all-male focus group of youths between the ages of 15 and 18 articulated a number of perceptions regarding condoms garnered from abstinence education in schools and church groups. Almost all of the participants felt condoms were unreliable as HIV/AIDS protection and, moreover, that they encouraged promiscuity (Flint 2009f, 2009g, 2009h). These two points are endorsed by many faith-based groups, including the Catholic Church (Lòpez Trujillo 2003). A meta-analysis of 174 studies, published in the *Journal of Acquired Immune Deficiency Syndromes* similarly found that:

> Evaluation of the influence of condom-related intervention features on ... outcomes of interest [that] indicated that ... increased numbers of sexual occasions, larger numbers of partners, and more likely sexual activity are not iatrogenic effects of providing condoms or training in condom use skills and interpersonal negotiation skills (Smoak *et al* 2006).

Given the scepticism with which young people can view condoms – complaints include reduced sensation and the view that 'you can't eat a sweet with the wrapper on' (Flint 2009g) – it is potentially dangerous to allow conceptions pertaining to efficacy to go unchallenged. This was a point emphasized by the US Government's Accountability Office in 2006:

> The [Office of the U.S. Global AIDS Coordinator] OGAC's ABC guidance and the abstinence-until-marriage spending requirement, including OGAC's policies for implementing it, have presented challenges for country teams. First, although most teams found the ABC guidance generally clear, two-thirds reported that ambiguities in some parts of the guidance led to uncertainty about implementing the model ... Second, although several teams told GAO that they value the ABC model and emphasize AB messages for certain populations, teams also reported that the spending requirement can limit their efforts to design prevention programs that are integrated and responsive to local prevention needs (GAO 2006).

It is difficult to decide the extent of the controversy; whilst abstinence/fidelity programmes certainly form an integral part of PEPFAR, they consume a relatively small proportion of the overall budget. In the 2008 financial year, only 7.4 percent of a total of $6 billion was set aside for this purpose (PEPFAR 2009c). (Although the relative accumulated socio-cultural impact of this minimal expenditure may prove to be disproportionately high.) The overwhelming majority of PEPFAR funds are devoted to treatment, not prevention. However, prevention initiatives are an extremely important component of any attempt to combat HIV/AIDS and undermining 'best practice' on the basis of ideology is questionable to say the least.

Much of the PEPFAR budget is targeted at treating HIV/AIDS sufferers, with 49 percent of Financial Year 2008 funding earmarked for such treatment (PEPFAR 2009c). However, another early criticism of the PEPFAR regime was its general insistence on the use of branded drugs. Taking into account the price disparities between branded and generic medicines, this approach generated a significant degree of criticism. The argument proffered by opponents was that more effective use could have been made of these monies had cheaper generic medicines been utilized instead. Given the advances made by firms producing generic drugs, in 2004 the US Government's Accountability Office highlighted the potential for improving the rollout of ARVs to sufferers:

> Since 2000, the price of ARV drugs has dropped considerably, from a high of more than $10,000 per person per year to a few hundred dollars or less per person annually, owing in part to the increased availability of generic ARV drugs and public pressure (GAO 2004).

Despite the obvious economic benefits of cost reduction, in the early years of PEPFAR only branded drugs were authorized for distribution. The rationale was that only branded drugs had been approved by a 'stringent regulatory authority' (GAO 2004). Only a regulatory body such as the US Food and Drug Administration (FDA), it was argued, could demonstrate the necessary levels of safety and efficacy. The result was that, by 2005, only 5 percent of the budget set aside for ARVs was spent on generics (Ismail 2005), despite the fact that many generics had been accepted onto the World Health Organization's prequalified list.[1] There was also disquiet when Randall Tobias, a former Chief Executive of pharmaceutical giant Eli Lilly, was in 2003 appointed by Bush as Global AIDS Co-ordinator with responsibility for PEPFAR. Critics saw the move as indicative of the power and reach of 'Big Pharma'. However, these fears were allayed somewhat when legislation passed in 2004 enabled the 'fast tracking' of HIV/AIDS drugs through the FDA. Atripla, a fixed-dose combination tablet was granted approval in just three months – this in comparison to traditional test periods of, sometimes, more than a year (FDA 2006). By the end of 2008, 78 AIDS-related generic medicines had been approved or 'tentatively' approved by the body (PEPFAR 2009c). Even prior to this, in 2007, nearly three quarters of ARVs being distributed by PEPFAR were generics, an estimated saving of $64 million (PEPFAR 2008). At the same time, the majority of these generics are first-line ARVs. Second-line ARVs remain expensive and the majority of approved drugs in this category remain branded (see Chapter 8 for a discussion on issues pertaining to branded/generic drugs and second-line therapies).

Research in the *Annals of Internal Medicine* in 2009 showed the results of a quantitative study into PEPFAR's effectiveness (Bendavid and Bhattacharya 2009). The study compared the 12 PEPFAR-funded African states with a 'control group' of 29 other African countries experiencing generalized HIV/AIDS epidemics over a ten year period from 1997 to 2007. It considered HIV/AIDS trends both prior to and subsequent to the implementation of PEPFAR. Prevalence rates amongst adults aged 15 to 49, deaths linked to HIV/AIDS and the number of adults living with HIV/AIDS were targeted as basic indicators in the survey. The results were somewhat mixed. In terms of HIV prevalence, there was no difference between the annual growth rates in either the focus or control countries. Likewise, the evidence seems to suggest that growth rates in the number of people living with HIV/AIDS was not significantly slower in the focus countries during the time in which PEPFAR was rolled out. However, the data linked to death rates from HIV/AIDS provide a more positive picture for PEPFAR. Following the implementation of PEPFAR, death rates from HIV/AIDS declined far more rapidly in the focus countries, the difference in the percentage change being 10.5 points lower in these countries compared to 3.5 percent lower in the control countries (Bendavid and Bhattacharya 2009). The study argues that the decline in the HIV/AIDS death rates is 'probably' the result of increased access to ARVs, the purchase and distribution of which account for nearly 50 percent of PEPFAR expenditure. According to these figures, PEPFAR has succeeded in averting 1.2 million deaths (2004–2007).

Framing HIV/AIDS as a security threat: The Clinton administration

What stands out immediately about PEPFAR is the sheer scale of the funding available, which, as mentioned, is unprecedented in terms of development spending. What is interesting is how American policymakers managed to generate the requisite levels of domestic support. There are striking differences between the Clinton and Bush administrations' framing of the HIV/AIDS debate and their subsequent ability to mobilize both people and resources in order to target the pandemic. For the Clinton administration, HIV/AIDS was understood in terms of security, while the Bush administration shifted the terms of the debate off the security agenda, onto a less tangible religious and moral framework. The Clinton security framework suggests a more significant prioritization of resources and executive attention for HIV/AIDS, but, in reality, this was not the case. It was the Bush approach that resulted in the more dramatic increase in funding and, more importantly, political commitment. It seems counter-intuitive that PEPFAR, based less on US 'national security interests' and motivated more by a largely moral, Christian worldview, could be so successful in the mobilization of such a landmark response. That so much funding was mobilized despite the lack of any apparent gains for US interests seems at odds with the perceived 'neoconservative' Bush agenda. However it is clear that the Bush response to HIV/AIDS in sub-Saharan Africa was highly reflective of the prevailing neoconservative thought that so shaped American foreign policy following the seismic events of 2001.

In the 1980s and early 1990s, HIV/AIDS in sub-Saharan Africa was viewed as a basic health and development issue (Elbe 2006). The debate was reframed in the mid- to late 1990s, when the Clinton White House began to explicitly link HIV/AIDS to the global security agenda. This change in focus formed part of an increasingly prevalent view amongst intellectuals and policymakers that what constituted 'security' needed to be expanded to incorporate a far broader agenda. In 1991, Clinton, not yet president, argued that 'our definition of security must include common threats to all people. On the environment and other global issues, our very survival depends upon the United States taking the lead' (Clinton 1991). During this period, alongside the looming possibility of the outbreak of 'water wars', environmental degradation as a security issue received a considerable degree of academic attention. The possibility of escalating 'resource conflicts' was assessed in great detail by Thomas Homer-Dixon (1994) and other members of the Project on Environment, Population and Security at the University of Toronto (Gleick 1992; Lowi 1992; Suhrke 1993) as part of the growing post-Cold War interest in 'non-traditional security threats'.

The post-Cold War reframing of HIV/AIDS was reflected in a range of speeches and policy documents emanating from the Clinton White

House. HIV/AIDS was consistently linked to the security interests of both the US and the wider international community. The securitization of HIV/AIDS is arguably articulated most clearly in the heavily US-influenced United Nations Security Council Resolution 1308 (SCR 1308) of 2000, in which the UN Security Council can be seen:

> *Recognizing* that the spread of HIV/AIDS can have a uniquely devastating impact on all sectors and levels of society,
> *Reaffirming* the importance of a coordinated international response to the HIV/AIDS pandemic, given its possible growing impact on social instability and emergency situations,
> *Further recognizing* that the HIV/AIDS pandemic is also exacerbated by conditions of violence and instability, which increase the risk of exposure to the disease through large movements of people, widespread uncertainty over conditions, and reduced access to medical care,
> *Stressing* that the HIV/AIDS pandemic, if unchecked, may pose a risk to stability and security.

The UN Security Council resolution can be viewed as the culmination of the Clinton government's attempts to explicitly link HIV/AIDS to security. Previously, in 1996, a Presidential Decision Directive described HIV/AIDS, together with a number of other diseases like Ebola and drug-resistant tuberculosis, as being 'one of the most significant health and security challenges' to face the international community (US Government 1996). Likewise, in 1999, HIV/AIDS was described by the White House as one of a range of 'transnational security threats' emanating from 'pockets of Africa' (US Government 1999). In 2000, the CIA issued a report on 'The Global Infectious Disease Threat and its Implications for the United States' in which it was argued that diseases like HIV/AIDS would 'complicate US and global security over the next 20 years', potentially undermining other developing regions (National Intelligence Council 2000). The framing of HIV/AIDS in this manner led Clinton, in late April 2000, to categorize the disease as a threat to 'national security' (Johnson 2002). It was during the same period that the United Nations Security Council, in an unprecedented move, also discussed HIV/AIDS as a threat to international security alongside the other non-traditional security threats of environmental degradation and terrorism (UN 2000). This discussion led to the Security Council adopting Resolution 1308 and, in 2002, establishing the Global Fund.

However, while the securitization of an issue by the White House would under normal circumstances entail a prioritization of resources and executive attention, under Clinton – the rhetoric notwithstanding – this was not the case. Despite the unparalleled focus on disease as a matter of US and international security during the late 1990s, this new aspect of the securitization agenda provoked a somewhat underwhelming response from both Congress and the administration itself. Funding to combat HIV/AIDS in Africa began to rise steadily but unspectacularly: from $51 million and $63 million in FY1998 and FY1999 respectively (Copson 2003), to $100 million for FY 2000 and FY2001 respectively (USAID 2000). The increase in government funding was accompanied by a similar increase in private sector funding, with the billionaire founder of Microsoft, Bill Gates, *via* the auspices of his Bill and Melinda Gates Foundation (2001), pledging $100 million at the annual World Economic Forum in Davos in 2001.[2] However, to put these sums into perspective, in 2000, the UN estimated that sub-Saharan Africa would need an annual commitment of approximately $4.6 billion in HIV/AIDS funding (Copson 2003).

Framing HIV/AIDS as a moral crusade: The Bush administration

The legacy of US President George W. Bush will arguably come to encompass the collapse of Enron, the 'War on Terror' invasions of Afghanistan and Iraq, and the sub-prime mortgage crisis and subsequent global recession. On leaving office in 2008, Bush's approval rating was just 24 percent; one of the lowest presidential approval ratings since this type of polling began (Jacobson 2009). What is frequently forgotten by supporters and critics alike is that during his presidency funding for HIV/AIDS prevention and treatment, under PEPFAR, reached unprecedented levels, dwarfing the efforts of the earlier, more overtly 'socially aware' Clinton administration. At the heart of the Bush administration's response to HIV/AIDS, over and above its framing in moral and/or religious terms, lies the notion of 'American exceptionalism'. The term, coined by Alexis de Tocqueville in his 1835 *Democracy in America*, proffers the idea of the US as a nation 'apart' given that its national identity is based, supposedly, on enlightenment ideals rather than race, language or culture. Historically, exceptionalism has informed American foreign policy. The notion of a 'manifest destiny' has arguably led to a 'doctrine that one nation has a preeminent social worth, a distinctively lofty mission, and consequently, unique rights in the application of moral principles' (Weinberg in Zinn 1990). It remains a recurring theme in American politics and is especially true of the neoconservativism that dominated the Bush Presidency, reaching its high point with the invasion of Saddam Hussein's Iraq in 2003. American exceptionalism has come to pivot on the idea that America should use its position as the world's only superpower to adjudicate issues of right and wrong, enforce order and essentially operate above the level of the international community (Ikenberry 2004). Furthermore, it is a project based on the potential implementation of American leadership and unilateralism. PEPFAR should be viewed as an extension of this worldview.

The rationale for the Democrat focus on non-traditional security threats was based on the idea that in the post-Cold War era increasing global interconnectivity would shape security concerns and responses. Even prior to the destruction of the World Trade Centre in 2001, the new Republican administration saw non-traditional security threats in a very different way, with the soon-to-be Deputy Secretary of Defence, Paul Wolfowitz, writing in 2000 that 'what is wrong with these claims is not that AIDS in Africa or the environment are not serious problems; rather it is the implication that conventional security is no longer something we need to worry much about' (cited in Hirsh 2003). The view from the new Bush administration was that while HIV/AIDS in regions like sub-Saharan Africa was undoubtedly a serious issue for the international community, it was not a matter of 'national security'. This different approach to 'framing' the debate on HIV/AIDS helped to shape PEPFAR as an initiative far less closely linked to a security agenda.

George W. Bush did not abandon entirely the rhetoric of HIV/AIDS as a security threat. HIV/AIDS was referenced in both the 2002 and 2006 National Security Strategies, albeit not couched directly in the language of the previous administration; documents emanating from Bush's office were far more circumspect in this regard (US Government 2002, 2006). Bush himself also articulated the view that HIV/AIDS had the potential to exacerbate the conditions necessary to bring about failed states (US Government 2008a). However, there is no doubt that morality and 'American exceptionalism' played a far greater role in shaping the Bush administration's response to HIV/AIDS. In anticipation of the 2007 World AIDS Day, Bush made clear his view that the US should use its superpower status as a 'force for good' (US Government 2007), describing his administration's commitment to fighting HIV/AIDS as a 'work of mercy', on a number of occasions (US Government 2003b, 2003e, 2008b). Such utterances built on claims made in 2003, at the time that PEPFAR was authorized, that the initiative was a 'great mission of rescue', and echoed President Woodrow Wilson's claim that 'America has a spiritual energy in her which no other nation can contribute to the liberation of mankind' (US Government 2003c).

Bush's framing of PEPFAR was frequently overtly religious. The President regularly employed terms such as 'redemption' and 'healing' (US Government 2007) when discussing PEPFAR, referring to America's mission as a response to a 'higher calling' (US Government 2008a). Other religiously-motivated justifications abound. In a 2004 speech in Philadelphia, Bush alluded to PEPFAR with the biblical reference that 'to whom much has been given, much is demanded' (US Government 2004). Such sentiments were echoed in, for example, a speech made prior to his five-nation tour of Africa in 2008 (Benin, Ghana, Liberia, Rwanda, Tanzania), during which he argued that 'we're all children of God, and having the power to save lives comes with the obligation to use it' (US Government 2008b).

Bush's framing proved far more potent in mobilizing the American response to the pandemic than Clinton's appeal to a broadened conception of security. The US public were never entirely convinced by the rhetoric of an African pandemic as a threat to national security. Neither were the majority of politicians. However, the notion that America had a moral responsibility to respond to HIV/AIDS outwith its own borders proved extremely powerful in drawing together and motivating elements that had previously looked upon it as a disease with negative moral connotations.

When discussing PEPFAR and HIV/AIDS, Bush made frequent references to America's special position in global politics and its obligation to use its power and influence for altruistic purposes. At the enactment of PEPFAR in May 2003, Bush declared that 'America makes this commitment for a clear reason, directly rooted in our founding. We believe in the value and dignity of every human life' (US Government 2003d). In the same speech he continued: 'the United States of America has the power and we have the moral duty to help. And I'm proud that our blessed and generous nation is fulfilling that duty'. Similar claims were made in subsequent speeches, with Bush arguing that 'this spirit of purpose and compassion has always defined America' (US Government 2008a) and that PEPFAR was inspired by 'the generosity of the American people. We are a nation of compassionate and good-hearted folks' (US Government 2008b).

PEPFAR under the Obama administration

Given the strong moral underpinnings of PEPFAR, with its emphasis on abstinence education and faith-based organizations, secular critics and non-faith-based HIV/AIDS organizations were heartened by Barack Obama's election as US President in November 2008. Obama (2008), in a speech on World AIDS Day in January 2006, had already alluded to some concerns regarding PEPFAR's overtly ideological ethos:

> We are all sick because of AIDS – and we are all tested by this crisis. It is a test not only of our willingness to respond, but of our ability to look past the artificial divisions and debates that have often shaped that response. When you go to places like Africa and you see the problem up close, you realise that it's not a question of treatment or prevention – or even what kind of prevention – it is all of the above. It is not an issue of either science or values – it is both. Yes, there must be more money spent on this disease. But there must also be a change in hearts and minds, in cultures and attitudes. Neither philanthropist nor scientist, neither government nor church, can solve this problem on their own – AIDS must be an all-hands-on-deck effort.

In his campaign literature, Obama (2008) took pains to stress the importance of prevention strategies that were based on 'sound science' and best practice, rather than moral predetermination. Likewise, while his campaign literature argued in favour of the reauthorization of PEPFAR, it highlighted the need to rewrite the ideological approach of the plan (Obama 2008). As a result, since Obama became president, there has been a degree of concern regarding the future of PEPFAR. It is possible that funding might 'flat-line' at 2009 levels. In May 2009, Obama asked the US Congress to approve the funding of $63 billion, to be targeted at global health over the following six years (PEPFAR 2010). The Obama administration's plan was to devote $51 billion to HIV/AIDS, malaria and tuberculosis over six years instead of five, which despite Obama's election pledge to significantly increase funding in this area, equated to a 2009-level funding 'freeze'. The fact that Obama ignited a partisan row over the provision of domestic healthcare services, together with the reality that there is evidence that many Americans had come to believe that their country was already doing all that it could where HIV/AIDS in sub-Saharan Africa was concerned, means that plans for the expansion of PEPFAR may inevitably be affected.

HIV/AIDS: A *cause célèbre*?

PEPFAR, Global Fund and MAP are illustrative of the fact that the international community has begun to take HIV/AIDS seriously. Despite the unprecedented level of funding currently offered by PEPFAR, the Global Fund and MAP, critics maintain that this is still simply not enough. In

2005, UNAIDS called for a significant increase in funding, estimating, post-2008, the need for expenditure in excess of $20 billion per year (UNAIDS 2005). 2009 projections suggested that for 2010, $25.1 billion would be required for low- and middle-income countries (UNAIDS 2009b). This was to ensure that 6.7 million people had access to ARVs, that 70 million pregnant women would be screened for HIV and that over eight billion condoms would be distributed. Based on this level of support, 2.6 million new infections would be prevented and 1.3 million deaths prevented (UNAIDS 2009b).

At the same time, there is a significant degree of debate as to whether the current HIV/AIDS funding models are appropriate. There is a case for arguing that too much funding is being targeted specifically at HIV/AIDS. In 2007, an article appeared in the *British Medical Journal* entitled 'Are we spending too much on HIV?' (England 2007). It caused a storm of controversy. The author, Roger England, argued that HIV/AIDS has absorbed a disproportionate degree of healthcare funding: in 2004, 21 percent of global health aid was spent on HIV/AIDS. In sub-Saharan Africa, 40 percent of all health aid was spent on HIV/AIDS. England suggested that, by 2010, HIV/AIDS would absorb nearly half of annual health aid – a figure arguably inconsistent with the severity of its impact (England 2007). England argued that spending on HIV/AIDS is ineffective relative to the costs associated with combating malaria, childhood illnesses, and tuberculosis. The funding set aside for combating HIV/AIDS would have a more immediate impact if, for example, it were used to purchase bed nets to prevent malaria. He argued that HIV/AIDS campaigners had been instrumental in turning the disease into a *cause célèbre* and, in so doing, had created an 'AIDS industry' which obscured the extent of the overall healthcare crisis in sub-Saharan Africa (Chapter 1):

> One factor surely has been the success of HIV lobbies and activists in promoting HIV as exceptional. In rich countries, HIV has become the crusade of the famous, fashionable, and influential. ... The exceptional status accorded HIV, and its excessive relative funding, has produced the biggest vertical programme in history, with its own staff, systems, and structure. This is having deleterious effects apart from underfunding of other diseases. ... National AIDS commissions, country coordinating mechanisms, UN agencies, etc are tripping over each other for funds and influence (England 2007).

England argued that instead of targeting a single disease, donors should concentrate on developing healthcare systems in developing countries that have the capacity and capability to deal with a spectrum of health-related issues. While controversial, his has been by no means a lone voice and his view has been echoed in a report for the Centre for Global Development that questions the overall efficacy of channelling significant resources into the combating of a single disease (Oomman *et al* 2008). The report argued that the single biggest impediment to improved healthcare in sub-Saharan Africa was a shortage of healthcare professionals (Oomman *et al* 2008). The dearth of qualified practitioners is arguably due to poor salaries, the lack of any inducement to commit long term to the sector and little prospect of performance-related job enhancement. By failing to concentrate on enhancing capacity, the rollout of ARVs has in some instances been heavily curtailed. In Uganda, stored consignments of donor-purchased drugs expired for want of an effective distribution network (Nakkazi 2006). There is therefore a clear-cut argument in favour of a shift away from HIV/AIDS as a 'special case' towards a new focus on aid that prioritizes healthcare in general.

Could PEPFAR funding be better spent? A continued focus on PEPFAR, even if, under the Obama administration it becomes somewhat financially diluted, may serve simply to skew US policy on Africa away from other issues of equal importance: state-building, primary education, the rule of law and increased economic growth. It is arguable that if Africa is to achieve real stability and prosperity, then the underlying causes of the continuing 'African Crisis' must be addressed (Prendergast and Norris 2009). Concentrating the bulk of foreign aid on African HIV/AIDS will not address the instability in, for instance, the DRC, Somalia and Sudan, which has claimed millions of lives. Difficult though a decision to 'abandon' HIV/AIDS might be, the prioritization of efforts to stabilize such conflicts might well be the best way forward. HIV/AIDS, by this reckoning, is a symptom of a wider malaise. In his efforts to address the 'African Crisis', Obama, with his African ancestry, has an opportunity to sidestep accusations of neo-imperialism in his dealings with African states in a way that would never have been possible for a president like George W. Bush. Obama is therefore well-placed to implement changes that, for all their short-term disadvantages, may well effect the best possible long-term results for sub-Saharan Africa.

However, it is precisely the high profile of HIV/AIDS that has generated these levels of funding and, in the case of PEPFAR, its moral imperative. While arguments in favour of increased healthcare generally certainly do have their merits, history suggests that it is unlikely that such a call to arms would provide a catalyst for increased funding levels. There is always the possibility that moral fervour might wane in the face of global

economic hardship. Following 2000, the Bush administration dramatically increased overseas development assistance, with the bulk of this
funding aimed at the reconstruction of Afghanistan and Iraq and the
combating of HIV/AIDS. In 2007, funding for HIV/AIDS in sub-Saharan
Africa accounted for nearly 23 percent of US aid to the region. In comparison, funding for other development programmes increased only mar-
ginally (Radelet *et al* 2008). However, the 2008 global economic recession,
a weak dollar and the cost of the US occupation of Afghanistan and Iraq,
have begun to place a considerable restraint on US aid to developing
countries. In recent years, there has been a trend towards declining levels
of US overseas development assistance, from $27.9 billion in 2005 to
$21.8 billion in 2007 (Radelet *et al* 2008). If inflation is accounted for in
the equation, then this fall represents a 26 percent decline in two years.
Under such a scenario 'something has to give' and less high-profile non-
HIV/AIDS lines of development funding might suffer.

Conclusion

Although funding for HIV/AIDS treatment and prevention has increased
dramatically over the past decade, the initial response of the international
community was relatively slow. While funding levels now reflect how
seriously HIV/AIDS is perceived as a development issue, the fact that there
are competing agencies operating in this sphere potentially undermines
the good to which this funding might be put. The three key players in
combating the disease in sub-Saharan Africa, PEPFAR, the Global Fund
and MAP, have adopted contrasting approaches in this regard. PEPFAR
stands out both in terms of the scale of its funding and in its unilateral
approach. Given its quasi neo-imperialist perspective, PEPFAR can in
many respects be viewed as a throwback to another age of development
politics. The presidency of George W. Bush was not without its critics,
indelibly linked as it was to a neoconservative agenda that prioritized the
US as a moral force in global politics. It is arguable that Bush's presidency
epitomized the arrogance inherent in the notion of 'American exceptionalism', with the war in Iraq representing a nadir in US foreign policy and
neoconservative aspirations for a 'new American century' (see the 'neo-
con' Project for the New American Century website as an articulation of
this cosmology – http://www.newamericancentury.org). However, it was
this same sense of 'mission' that drove the creation of PEPFAR and its
accompanying, unprecedented levels of funding. If Clinton's efforts to
frame HIV/AIDS as a security issue did little to galvanize the American
public behind the fight against HIV/AIDS, in framing HIV/AIDS as a

moral issue, Bush succeeded in creating a momentum behind efforts to stay the pandemic, bringing on board the American religious right – a group that had traditionally viewed HIV/AIDS as a disease of promiscuity and moral degeneration. By concentrating on America's moral obligation to be a 'force for good' in world politics, Bush succeeded in persuading Congress to authorize, in 2008, $48 billion for HIV/AIDS in Africa. At the same time, it was exactly this 'moral mission' that also generated some of the more controversial elements inherent in PEPFAR; in particular, its focus on abstinence education for young people as the basis for its prevention strategy. Allegations that the initiative was driven by 'ideology', rather than best practice, were frequently levelled at PEPFAR policymakers. Furthermore, the unilateral approach adopted by the American government with respect to the implementation of PEPFAR and its preference for working with faith-based organizations, together with fears concerning the influence of 'Big Pharma', made for negative headlines in the early days of the programme. Many of these fears have been subsequently allayed; unilateralism has resulted in an effective disbursement of funds, generic ARVs are now a staple of PEPFAR's rollout of drugs to HIV/AIDS sufferers, the FDA has been reconfigured to approve HIV/AIDS-related medicines far more quickly and the government's position on abstinence-only education, whilst still contentious, has softened since 2003.

Two significant – and mutually opposed – criticisms remain, the first being that global HIV/AIDS spending remains insufficient (and may even be decreasing) and the second, that HIV/AIDS is being funded to levels disproportionate to other equally pressing issues pertaining to the 'African Crisis': failed states, civil conflict, instability, poverty and poor governance. There is something to be said for both arguments, although if other developed countries followed the US' lead then the question of funding would arguably become mute. Evidence that 1.2 million deaths have been averted through the timely provision of ARVs represents a clear demonstration that PEPFAR has been effective. Although Obama's flat-lining of funding has raised questions about his commitment to PEPFAR, his commitment to moving away from the 'ideological' stance of the Bush era, towards a focus on prevention strategies based on best practice, appears to have quelled critics concerned with the impact and efficacy of morality-based interventions. However, the international response to HIV/AIDS must also be considered in broader international terms.

7
Morality, Behavioural Change and the Search for a 'Social Vaccine'

In the absence of an HIV/AIDS vaccine, and against a complex socio-political and economic backdrop, endeavours to formulate a successful strategy to stay the HIV/AIDS pandemic in sub-Saharan Africa have varied considerably. At one end of the spectrum lie responses based on faith – either traditional Christian or Islamic values of sexual morality or in similarly traditional African medicine (Chapter 5), all of which can be at odds with the Western biomedical approach. Largely successful efforts by Western governments to counter the spread of HIV/AIDS amongst homosexual populations in the US and Europe have tended to focus on the disease as a medical issue. Efforts have concentrated on interventions that reduce the chance of exposure by those most at risk of contracting HIV/AIDS. Campaigns centring on the use of condoms and 'safer-sex' have been hallmarks of such drives. However, as the rampant spread of HIV/AIDS during the past three decades attests, the safer-sex approach has been notably less successful in sub-Saharan Africa, prompting calls for a re-examination of the safer-sex model's suitability for the region. In particular, Christian faith-based organizations (FBOs) have long pressed for an alternative approach based on a focus on behavioural change, in effect a 'social vaccine'. There are an estimated 495 million Christians in sub-Saharan Africa, making Christianity the largest religion on the continent, followed closely by Islam, which has 420 million adherents (WRD 2008). Geographically, while Islam is influential in many parts of sub-Saharan Africa, particularly in countries like Nigeria and Senegal, the majority of adherents live to the north of the continent. Muslim groups have been active in the fight against the pandemic. However, greater funding (especially post-PEPFAR[1] – Chapter 6), continental reach and influence have resulted in Christian FBOs and religiously-motivated individuals having a more significant impact on the shaping of behavioural change in the region.

The concept of behavioural change as a 'social vaccine' is problematic from a Western 'rights' perspective through which proponents endeavour not to judge individuals for their sexual or lifestyle choices. The faith-based model, which encompasses clear proscriptions against promiscuity and homosexuality in the interests of heterosexual fidelity, runs counter to liberal ideals of personal freedom and choice. Given that the Western model developed out of the experience of treating and educating largely homosexual populations, this is unsurprising. It is equally unsurprising that established AIDS charities, often with a largely homosexual membership base in Europe and America, have reacted angrily to what groups like the International Gay and Lesbian Human Rights Commission (IGLHRC) perceive to be a 'hijacking' of the HIV/AIDS agenda in sub-Saharan Africa by the American religious right (Johnson 2007). The matter of a 'social vaccine' is also tied to issues of 'traditional values'. As discussed in Chapter 1, the spread of diseases such as syphilis during the colonial area were blamed, in some quarters, on the erosion of traditional safeguards governing sexuality, particularly the sexuality of African women (Lambkin 1914). Similarly, the inherently conservative social agenda accompanying many morality-driven campaigns in sub-Saharan Africa centred on sexual behaviour aims to 'protect' society from pernicious outside influences that could potentially undermine the community fabric. For secular AIDS activists, particularly in the early days of the pandemic in Africa, engaging with religious groups in order to fight the disease meant a moral dilemma. For secularists, the prioritization of 'sexual morality' issues by faith communities meant that it was difficult to escape the conclusion that campaigns by religious groups and associated FBOs had a dual agenda; there was always the possibility that 'best practice' might be ignored in favour of faith-based tenets.

Strategies targeting risk reduction and behavioural change became the foci of an increasingly bitter debate that is yet to be resolved adequately. At the heart of the debate lies Uganda, Africa's one apparent success story in the fight against HIV/AIDS. Uganda's success, proponents claim, came about as a result of 'behavioural changes' encouraged by the country's evangelical 'born-again' Christian President Yoweri Museveni. The strategy encompassed three core elements: abstinence before marriage, fidelity and an emphasis on 'traditional values'. The 'Ugandan miracle' has been deconstructed enthusiastically by policymakers – particularly those linked to the PEPFAR programme – in the interests of extrapolating its 'formula' to neighbouring states. Critically, much future policymaking is potentially dependent on the veracity of the Ugandan experience, particularly in light of the considerable funding opportunities that have been on offer as a result of US largesse. Using Uganda as a case study, this chapter considers the impact of FBOs and religiously-motivated individuals in shaping an alternative HIV/AIDS prevention paradigm based on moral values and behavioural change.

Healthcare provision by faith-based groups

In many African countries, faith-based groups have been second only to governments in the provision of healthcare and education. In 2005, a Global Health Council (2005) report estimated that in poorer countries faith-based groups provided as much as 40 percent of all healthcare. Furthermore, away from urban centres, such groups are frequently the only source of credible medical care. The Catholic Church is a good case in point. Catholic agencies operating under the umbrella of *Caritas Internationalis*, a confederation of Catholic charities, are active in 107 countries worldwide, 33 of which are in Africa, providing and operating over 5,000 hospitals and nearly 18,000 dispensaries (Caritas 2008). Catholic Relief Services (CRS), the humanitarian agency established by the Catholic Church in America, supplies ARV drugs to 84,000 people while taking care of a further 150,000 not yet prescribed such treatment (CRS 2008a). The vast majority of these beneficiaries live in Africa.[2] In Malawi, the Medical Missionaries of Mary has established a healthcare network covering 76 rural villages (MMM 2008). Even in South Africa, the wealthiest country on the continent, the Catholic Church is, after the government, the second-largest provider of care for those infected with HIV/AIDS. CRS (2008a), over and above providing practical care to sufferers, has also published material on HIV/AIDS 'best practice' and even 'promising practice', material that has been made readily available to other agencies and actors. The Anglican Church (2008), with nearly 80 million members, is the third-largest Christian domination in the world after the Catholic and Russian Orthodox Churches respectively. It, too, plays a significant role in shaping HIV/AIDS policy and treatment in much of Africa.

Many secular groups operating in the field are uncomfortable about the proselytizing opportunities potentially available to faith-based groups involved in HIV/AIDS work. At the same time, the fact remains that these groups are all but indispensable in much of sub-Saharan Africa, as was duly noted by a World Bank study of healthcare in Uganda in 2003:

> religious not-for-profit facilities are more likely to provide pro-poor services and services with a public good element, and charge strictly lower prices for services than for-profit units. Faith-based not-for-

profit and for-profit facilities both provide better quality care than their government counterparts, although government facilities have better equipment. These findings are consistent with there being a premium in working in a religious not-for-profit facility and that religious not-for-profits are driven (partly) by altruistic concerns ... working for God appears to matter (Reinikka and Svensson 2003).

A survey of 'key informants', including NGO workers, aid-agency personnel, healthcare professionals and politicians working in the area of HIV/ AIDS, conducted by the Global Health Council (2005) in Kenya, South Africa and Uganda, demonstrates that FBOs engaged in HIV/AIDS care are generally viewed in a positive light by the public. Respondents cited the ability of FBOs to mobilize at grassroots level, the high level of esteem in which they are held by local communities and their moral authority as instrumental in the fight against the pandemic; even the poorest and most remote of rural African locations tend to have a church of some description. Nevertheless, secular informants for the survey repeatedly raised concerns about overt proselytizing that it was felt could con-tribute to the ongoing stigmatization of AIDS sufferers (Global Health Council 2005).

Faith-based organizations and the fight against HIV/AIDS

FBOs may be controversial actors in the fight against HIV/AIDS, but their significance cannot be overstated. For example, globally, the Catholic Church alone is singularly responsible for nearly 27 percent of all centres that treat sufferers, a statistic that ensures its position as a key player (Lozano Barragán 2006). Furthermore, as critics have been eager to high-light, the Catholic Church has political power in its own right; the Vatican's status as a non-member permanent observer at the UN gives it an influence in the wording of any UN HIV/AIDS-related policy (HRW 2004). All of the major HIV/AIDS donors – including the World Health Organization, the United Nations and USAID – have acknowledged the importance of religious groups in the provision of care for those affected. The significance of FBOs was bolstered yet further with the establishment of the Bush administration's PEPFAR programme (Chapter 6) which, with an authorized budget of $48 billion for the period 2009–2013, afforded faith-based groups a prominent role in determining prevention strategies.

There are three key concerns that can be raised with regard to the potential consequences associated with FBO interventions: an emphasis on sexual morality and fidelity at the expense of 'safer-sex' education,

the increased stigmatization of victims by virtue of their 'moral culpability', and the reinforcement of traditional gender roles and gender
hierarchies. Since sexual morality is a pivotal issue for adherents, the
issue of condom use has been particularly divisive. The Catholic Church
in particular has come under fire for its reticence to promote condom
usage, and much has been made of controversial statements emanating
from the Pontifical Council for the Family, established by Pope John
Paul II in 1981 to guide Catholics on issues including procreation, sex
education and abortion. Since its inception, the Council has made a
number of strongly-worded pronouncements on the 'evils' of condoms,
maintaining, amongst other points, that they offer little protection against
the transmission of HIV because they promote promiscuity and trivialize
sex. In 1996, in the publication *The Truth and Meaning of Human Sexuality*,
the Council argued that:

> it is necessary to correct the opinion put about by information cam-
> paigns based on so-called 'safe sex' and spreading protective means
> (condoms). This position, in itself contrary to morality, also turns out
> to be fallacious and ends up increasing promiscuity and free sexual
> activity through a false idea of safety. Objective and scientifically rigor-
> ous studies have shown the high percentage of the failure of these
> means (Pontifical Council for the Family 1996).

The head of the Council from 1991 until his death in 2008, Cardinal Lòpez
Trujillo (2003), a morally-conservative cleric from Columbia, remained
outspoken in his opposition to condoms, stating that 'responsible sexual
behaviour takes place only in conjugal love, assuming the responsibilities
of marriage as a reciprocal, exclusive and total self-giving of a man and a
woman in a community of love and life'. Rather more problematically, he
also argued that HIV could pass through 'pores' in condoms and that since
encouraging condom use would result in higher levels of promiscuity,
the associated result would be higher levels of HIV transmission (Lòpez
Trujillo 2003). In 2007, the Catholic Bishop of Mozambique, Archbishop
Francisco Chimoio, added fuel to the fire with statements, widely circulated in the British media, articulating his belief not only in the inability
of condoms to protect against HIV, but in the idea that 'there are two
countries in Europe ... making condoms with the virus, on purpose'
(*Guardian* 27/09/2007).

The views expressed above are not universal to the Church as a whole.
The Catholic Agency for Overseas Development (CAFOD) has argued
strongly that the debate surrounding the efficacy and desirability of con-

dom use in preventing the spread of HIV is overly simplistic, divisive and unhelpful (Smith *et al* 2004). Its Catholic affiliations notwithstanding, CAFOD has argued that condoms can be effective as part of a wider, behavioural change strategy. In a presentation to the International AIDS Conference in Bangkok in 2004, CAFOD stressed the futility of seeking 'magic bullet' solutions to multidimensional, complex issues. The paper emphasized that any 'strategy that enables a person to move from a higher risk activity towards the lower end of the risk continuum is a valid risk reduction strategy ... [A] risk reduction continuum is compatible with the theology and moral codes of Christian faith-based organizations as well as with sound health promotion principles' (Smith *et al* 2004).

Behavioural change versus risk reduction

Much of the debate between secular and non-secular groups centres on questions of prevention and, in particular, strategies favouring either behavioural change or risk reduction. Amongst secular groups there is scepticism that sexual behaviour can be readily influenced, and an associated conviction that any intervention that might mitigate the risk of infection – condoms, for example – must be promoted. Data published in medical and health journals like the *New England Journal of Medicine*, *Family Planning Perspectives*, *Social Science and Medicine* and *Studies in Family Planning* on the effectiveness of condoms in combating the spread of HIV/AIDS vary from a low of 69 percent to a high of 94 percent. However, the lower ranges reflect individuals who use condoms inconsistently, thereby lowering the mean. A systematic review of the medical literature, sponsored by UNAIDS, suggests that condoms provide approximately 90 percent protection when used properly and consistently, most failures coming from 'breakage, slippage, and improper use' (Hearst and Chen 2004). This figure is supported by the WHO, which has emphasized that in studies 'condoms were effective in protecting against transmission of HIV to women and men ... [a]lthough condoms are not 100 percent effective, partial protection can substantially reduce the spread of STIs within populations' (Holmes *et al* 2004). Where condom usage has been backed heavily, in developed world homosexual populations and in countries like Thailand, there has been a discernible drop in HIV transmission. In Thailand, the government's successful '100 percent programme', approved in 1991, mandated that all brothels enforce condom usage or risk sanction. While this programme was successful in its own right, it also had the unexpected consequence of discouraging men from engaging in commercial sex by forcing them to consider the possible effects of their behaviour, thereby curbing transmission rates yet further (UNAIDS 2000a). However, for condoms to be truly effective against HIV/AIDS in sub-Saharan Africa, these need to be readily available. This is not always the case, particularly in rural areas. If condom supplies are unreliable and as a result only used intermittently, then the benefits are unlikely to be pronounced (Hearst and Chen 2004).

In stark contrast to secular organizations, many FBOs argue that behavioural change messages represent a more effective way of countering HIV/AIDS. Core behavioural-change strategies include encouraging individuals to delay sexual debut and reduce their number of sexual partners, and the promotion of abstinence and fidelity. A 2003 paper funded by USAID cited evidence from three studies conducted in sub-Saharan Africa that suggested that behavioural change is in fact more effective than 'safer-sex' in curbing transmission rates (Green 2003). The paper argued that while condoms are important in preventing the spread of HIV/AIDS amongst those who cannot easily embrace behavioural change – sex workers, for example – these behaviours remain dangerous. Post-2003, the scales tipped in favour of those advocating behavioural change in sub-Saharan Africa. The Bush administration's ongoing PEPFAR initiative, introduced in 2003 and unprecedented in terms of funding, was from the outset strongly in favour of abstinence education for teenagers. George W Bush famously remarked that abstinence is 'the only 100 percent effective means of preventing pregnancy, HIV, and sexually-transmitted infections' (Bush 2004). When PEPFAR was enacted, the original commitment of $15 billion was allocated as follows: 55 percent for treatment, 15 percent for palliative care, 10 percent for orphans and children, and 20 percent for HIV/AIDS prevention. Of the funding for prevention, 33 percent was designated for abstinence-until-marriage programmes (US Government 2003a). Critically, the PEPFAR act stipulated clearly that funding was not to be used to provide or educate teenagers in the use of condoms. Material generated in 2005 but still available on the PEPFAR website at the time of writing (April 2010) was unequivocal:

> Abstinence until marriage programs are particularly important for young people, as approximately half of all new infections occur in the 15- to 24-year-old age group. Delaying first sexual encounter can have a significant impact on the health and well-being of adolescents and on the progress of the epidemic in communities. In many of the countries hardest hit by HIV/AIDS, sexual activity begins early and prior to marriage. Surveys show that, on average, slightly more than 40 percent of women in sub-Saharan Africa have had pre-

marital sex before age 20; among young men, sex before marriage is even more common ... abstaining from sexual activity is the most effective and only certain way to avoid HIV infection (PEPFAR 2005).

Secular critics (Cohen 2003; HRW 2005) have argued that PEPFAR has facilitated a 'hijacking' of the prevention agenda by FBOs and conservative forces. Unsurprisingly, considering the fiercely emotive nature of the debate, it is difficult to gain a clear picture of the precise value of abstinence programmes in actually reducing sexual activity amongst teenagers. The USAID-funded report aside, evidence, garnered mainly from studies undertaken in American schools, is mixed (HRW 2002; Kay and Jackson 2008; Willcox 2008). In a 2008 paper sponsored by the US Department of Health and Human Services, 'A Scientific Review of Abstinence and Abstinence Programs', the University of Virginia sociologist Bradford Willcox has argued that abstinence initiatives have been successful. He has also argued that abstinence has improved immeasurably the lives of those influenced by the initiatives (Willcox 2008). Willcox's evidence is derived from a number of US studies purporting to demonstrate that teenagers who refrain from sex perform better at school and exhibit better mental and physical health than their non-abstaining counterparts:

Premarital sex, especially when initiated in early adolescence, seems to act as a gateway for some adolescents into problematic social networks and behaviours. Specifically, studies find that teenagers who engage in sex before marriage are more likely to be delinquent, to be addicted to alcohol or drugs, and to have problems in school, compared to their peers who abstain from having sex ... it seems likely that a majority of adolescents and adults (particularly females) who engage in premarital sex will experience at least one type of physical, psychological, social, or marital harm as a consequence of engaging in premarital sex (Willcox 2008).

Conversely, Julie F. Kay and Ashley Jackson (2008), in a paper sponsored by the Harvard School of Public Health, argue that those enrolled in abstinence programmes are just as likely to engage in sexual activity by the age of 16 as those who are not. General statistics suggest that the vast majority of Americans engage in premarital sex, with the average age of sexual debut being 17.4 years (Finer 2007). Kay and Jackson argue, too, that studies suggest that, when they do engage in intercourse, 'virginity pledgers' are less likely to use condoms, due partly to ambivalence as to their efficacy and partly to a lack of preparedness, thus exposing themselves to STIs and unplanned pregnancies. These findings augment an earlier Human Rights Watch survey into abstinence programmes undertaken in the US, which found that by continually emphasizing the limitations of condoms, such programmes actually put teenagers at risk by undermining their confidence in prophylactics as a form of protection against HIV/AIDS (HRW 2002). Abstinence as a normative strategy for sexual health is thus, at best, contentious.

Both sides of the 'safe-sex'/abstinence debate have argued that they have been deliberately undermined and constrained by funding bodies. CAFOD has contended that Global Fund monies have only been made available to organizations placing a heavy emphasis on condom usage and that UNAIDS has been unduly influenced by the pro-condom lobby (Smith *et al* 2004). Human Rights Watch has claimed the opposite, arguing that PEPFAR's influence has resulted in more funding being channeled towards pro-abstinence programmes (HRW 2005).

The 'Ugandan miracle'

Uganda has been seen to represent one of the few success stories in the fight against HIV/AIDS. The Ugandan HIV/AIDS 'model' is frequently upheld as 'best practice' for other African states. President Yoweri Museveni and his wife, Janet Museveni, both 'born-again' Christians, have become internationally renowned figures.[3] Evidence of Museveni's global stature was apparent during his tour of the US in November 2007, when he held meetings with key figures including George W. Bush, the then Secretary of State, Condeleezza Rice, and the Speaker of the House, Nancy Pelosi. Museveni's reputation rests upon an acknowledgement that his government successfully stayed the Ugandan HIV/AIDS pandemic and then proceeded to roll it back. Questions have, however, been raised as to the veracity of the Ugandan experience. Issues requiring reconsideration include the reliability of the data presented as evidence, actual evidence of behavioural change, Museveni's agenda, and the appropriation of the 'Ugandan miracle' by the American religious right.

Museveni was one of the first African leaders to accept the reality of his country's growing AIDS problem. He has argued that the seriousness of the pandemic was brought home to him during his first year in power, in 1986, when he was informed that 30 percent of a Ugandan military delegation sent to Cuba for training tested HIV-positive (Putzel 2004). The following year, in consultation with the WHO, the Ugandan government developed its AIDS Control Programme (ACP), the first of its kind in Africa. The government's approach was based on the 'ABC' system: A – abstinence, B – be faithful, C – use condoms. In an AIDS-related speech to the African Development Forum in December 2000, Museveni listed the achievements of his administration:

> As a result of our awareness campaign, close to 100 per cent [of Ugandans] know what HIV/AIDS is and how it is spread; the risks involved; and how it can be prevented. There are indications of positive behaviour change. Uganda's estimated prevalence rate reduced from around 30 per cent in the early 1990s to around 8 per cent in the late 1990s; the age of first sex among girls increased from 14 to 16 years; and from 14 to 17 among boys between 1995 and 1998; sex with non-regular partners has also considerably reduced; and condom use increased from 57.6 per cent in 1995 to 76 per cent in 1998. Next year, we shall require 80 million condoms. Most important of all, the stigma attached to people living with HIV/AIDS has virtually evaporated (Museveni 2000).

These were impressive achievements. Prevalence, which according to official figures for 1991 reached approximately 18 percent in rural areas and up to 30 percent in urban areas, had, in just ten years, declined to an average of between 6 and 7 percent nationwide (Ugandan Government 2008). A study for the Alan Guttmacher Institute – a left-leaning, 'pro-choice' US think-tank concerned with issues of sexual and reproductive health – demonstrated that, for the period 1988–2001, evidence for key behavioural changes amongst Ugandans was apparent (Singh *et al* 2003). The report contended that the government's ABC approach should be duly accredited with these changes. It found that over the course of the 1988–2001 period, there was evidence of an appreciable delay of almost nine months in sexual debut amongst girls of 15 to 17, that incidence of multiple sexual partners amongst Ugandans had declined, and that condom use had increased significantly. There was also evidence to suggest that the state had worked hard to ensure that HIV/AIDS was discussed at all levels of society, thereby decreasing ignorance and stigmatization.

However, there have been questions as to the extent of the 'Ugandan miracle'. Tim Allen (2005), of the London School of Economics, maintained that 'Uganda ... is like a cloud in which commentators see whatever shapes they fancy. Journalists, politicians and aid agency staff have become prone to exaggerate and dramatize, and this has clearly affected some of the more academic analysis too'. This situation can be partially explained by the lack of detailed, systematic data capable of providing an accurate 'snapshot' of the country as a whole. Ugandan HIV/AIDS statistics are by no means clear-cut and offer a significant degree of latitude with respect to interpretation. For example, little data are available from northern Uganda; incursions by the Lord's Resistance Army, a guerrilla group opposed to Museveni, have rendered much of the region ungovernable. In addition, there have been few concerted attempts to engage in controlled sampling; much of the data are derived from antenatal surveillance, which is not fully representative (Allen, T. 2005). Such uncertainty has arguably allowed both the Museveni administration and its critics to cherry-pick their statistics (Tumushabe 2006).

For all the government's concentration on behavioural change, the impressive drop in prevalence may have had little at all to do with government action. Prevalence levels can fall for two reasons, either a decline in infection rates or an increased mortality rate amongst those infected. In a controversial conference paper presented in 2005, Marie Wawer and her colleagues argued that high mortality rates alone could have accounted for five percentage points of Uganda's decline in prevalence to 2001 (Wawer *et al* 2005). In other words, the declining prevalence rate was a consequence of mortality rates outstripping infection rates (Wawer *et al* 2005). Wawer *et al* suggested that, rather than abstinence and monogamy, an increase in condom usage could explain the remainder of the declining prevalence. Tim Allen (2005), too, contended that as Uganda was one of the first countries to experience the disease the pandemic there was then in a far more 'mature' phase than it was in southern African countries, and that some form of 'natural levelling off' was inevitable.

Museveni's politicization of HIV/AIDS has enabled him to cement his position both as President and as a world leader in the fight against the pandemic. In a report for the UN Research Institute for Social Development, Joseph Tumushabe (2006) argued that Museveni has used his HIV/AIDS achievements to paper over the cracks in his administration. Tumushabe stressed how Museveni's post-2000 emphasis on Ugandan HIV/AIDS policies coincided with increased pressure on him to counter allegations of his government's economic mismanagement, corruption and oppression of opposition politicians. Museveni's rise as a global AIDS authority also redirected attention from his controversial 1997 decision to send the Ugandan army into the DRC to remove Joseph Mobutu from power, a decision that resulted in regional instability, the deaths of thousands of Congolese, and international condemnation of his administration.

Particularly post-2000, Museveni's faith-based approach won him both plaudits and vilification in almost equal measure. His increased emphasis on the merits of abstinence and fidelity over condom use caused considerable concern amongst those pressing for an increase in condom usage, particularly for teenagers. Critics dismissed his perspective as an attempt to curry favour with the Bush administration in the interests of securing funding and personal recognition.

Analysing the extent of behavioural change in Uganda

Museveni has justified his position on the basis of his religious convictions, his reverence for 'tradition' and his contempt for the 'corrosive' effects of Western secular values. With value-based norms forming the basis for Ugandan initiatives, therefore, it is necessary to evaluate the effects and efficacy of framing HIV/AIDS as a moral issue and to separate rhetoric from evidence, especially given that infection rates post-2001 are once again on the rise, albeit not dramatically.[4] George W Bush was lavish in his praise of Museveni and, consequently, Uganda was one of the chief beneficiaries of his PEPFAR initiative, with a budget allocation of $236 million in 2007, compared with $162 million for Mozambique and $103 million for Rwanda (PEPFAR 2009b). Of the African countries concerned, only South Africa, as befitting the country with the highest number of HIV infections, received more – an allocation of $397.8 million (PEPFAR 2009b). After meeting Museveni in New York City in September 2008, Bush declared that the former

> gave me great confidence when it came to realizing the proper strategy in dealing with HIV/AIDS, because of the success in Uganda that showed the rest of the continent and the rest of the world how strong leadership and a good strategy can actually save lives in a very substantial way (US Government 2008c).

Museveni (2004) has argued that by concentrating on abstinence and fidelity, a 'social vaccine' against the disease was engineered through deep-seated behavioural change and that, crucially, 'with no medical vaccine in sight ... this was within our modest means'. Controversially, the Musevenis have been reluctant to either champion condoms or ascribe any credit to 'safer-sex' programmes where Uganda's falling prevalence rates are concerned. The President is on record as describing condoms as 'un-African' and has also questioned their effectiveness in

HIV/AIDS prevention (Allen, T. 2005). Janet Museveni (2004) has argued that

> the truth is that there is no 'safe sex' outside of the situation of faith-fulness to a partner. Giving young people condoms is tantamount to giving them a license to go out and be promiscuous; it leads to certain death ... To encourage children to use condoms is to admit that you have no faith in the ability of human beings to make correct choices, once they are equipped with the right information.

In response to concerns about a potential condom shortage in 2004, the Ugandan government stated that it was not especially concerned about the availability of condoms and would instead be focusing on abstinence and behavioural-change campaigns (HRW 2005). At the XIV International Conference on AIDS and STDs held in Bangkok in 2004, Museveni made only passing reference to the value of condoms in the fight against HIV/AIDS, concentrating instead almost solely on abstinence and fidelity (Museveni 2004). Four years later, speaking to the major international aid and donor organizations including PEPFAR, Global Fund, the World Bank, WHO, UNAIDS and UNICEF, Museveni (2008) once again stressed that behavioural change, not condoms, was central to staying HIV/AIDS.

To a certain extent, Museveni's stance is credible. Surveys suggest that condom usage in Uganda, while on the rise, remains relatively low. In 1995, around the time that HIV-prevalence rates started to decrease, only 6 percent of Ugandan women had any familiarity with condoms. It there-fore appears unlikely that condom use alone can explain declining levels of HIV-prevalence during the 1990s (Hearst and Chen 2003). Such evid-ence has been used to validate the behavioural change approach, leading Museveni (2008) to ask:

> Uganda was among the lowest users of condoms and yet, it was in Uganda that there was this big decline in a very short time. So why? If behaviour change does not work, how does it happen that the low condom per capita users realized the very steep decline of HIV pre-valence? Why, in the countries, which had the much higher condom per capita use, we are experiencing real high rises of infection?

However, the Ugandan government's ambivalence toward condoms has had a number of profound effects. The 2004–2005 condom shortage in Uganda was caused by dwindling supplies of the domestic *Engabu* (Lugandan for 'shield') brand. Citing quality concerns, state officials withdrew millions of *Engabu* condoms from circulation. This withdrawal was significant because *Engabu* had been circulated free of charge and accounted for approximately 80 percent of all condoms distributed in Uganda (Bass 2005). Shortages were exacerbated by new state controls over condom imports, which were required to undergo additional domestic quality assessments before being released into circulation (Chattoe-Brown and Bitunda 2006). The resultant delays, together with a new government import duty on condoms destined for private sale, ensured that condoms rapidly became expensive, with the price rising ten-fold between October and December 2004 (Bass 2005). Even once pre-2004 circulation levels were restored, pro-condom campaigners were left fearing that the *Engabu* saga, which saw considerable media coverage about quality concerns, had created a lasting perception of condoms as unreliable in the fight against HIV/AIDS – an image that the government's lack of urgency regarding condom distribution did little to offset.

The evidence in favour of the behavioural change approach therefore remains unclear. Alternative explanations for Uganda's 'success' in tackling HIV/AIDS are available; a number of hypotheses which, like mortality rates outstripping infection rates, do not hinge on government policy, can account for the dramatic fall in prevalence between 1987 and 2001 (Wawer *et al* 2005). If government interventions are not responsible for the 'Ugandan miracle', then any attempts to replicate such policies elsewhere would be futile at best. Moreover, as will be argued below, behavioural change models can only be successful if individuals are actually able to dictate their behaviour. There is evidence to suggest that, in countries like Uganda, those whom abstinence programmes are designed to protect are the very ones at increased risk of infection; women in long-term relationships.

Gender hierarchies, behavioural change and risk reduction

The question of gender is an emotive but important element of the debate pertaining to HIV/AIDS programmes, both in Uganda in particular and in sub-Saharan Africa as a whole (Chapter 3). The issue of gender in the context of HIV/AIDS can be divided into two parts: division of labour, which determines the ability of women to act as independent agents, and cultural norms and values, which determine gender hierarchies. Key to engaging with both elements of this broader debate are notions of cultural relativity and cultural imperialism. Historically, especially during the colonial era, improved rights for women in Africa were blamed for providing the impetus for increased promiscuity and sexual immorality (Lambkin 1914; Fiedrich and Jellema 2003). Accusations of cultural insensitivity have bedevilled Western feminist theorists for decades. Feminist theorists themselves have struggled with this issue, questioning the 'cross-cultural effectiveness' of transposing western conceptions of gender to an African context (Higgins 2006). Western concepts of feminism are viewed with suspicion by many African elites, who consider them to be 'un-African' and a threat to the social fabric. Museveni has argued that imported western values undermine the sanctity of the family unit (Hanssen 2005). However, given that statistics show that women, especially young women, are disproportionately at risk of HIV infection, issues pertaining to gender cannot be pushed to one side in the interests of political correctness.

Both behavioural change and risk reduction strategies have been undermined by the inequalities thrown up by the gender divide in Uganda. Arguably, an emphasis on traditional values and fidelity has ensured that many women in Uganda have little control over their sexual behaviour. Unequal economic opportunity, combined with lower levels of education and conservative social norms, has served to make women dependent on men. Women's powerlessness is exacerbated by practices including polygamy, widow inheritance and female genital cutting. Marital rape is not illegal. When the Domestic Relations Bill (DRB) was outlined in Uganda in 2003, its adherents, backed by women's groups like the Uganda Women's Network, aimed to drive through measures that would strengthen the position of Ugandan women. However, questioning polygamy in particular threatened to derail the entire process. Ugandan Muslims reacted vociferously to plans to curtail it and, as a result, the Bill languished while a compromise was sought. It was eventually decided to break the Bill in two, with separate legislation for Muslims and non-Muslims. However, the resultant compromise has left many gender activists dissatisfied, given that key elements of the Bill, including marital rape, were seen to be sidelined. In 2008, one of the drafters of the Bill, Professor Joseph Kakooza, was questioned on the legality of marital rape:

There are grounds for refusing sex like after child birth, poor health condition after surgery, monthly periods or anything which makes it unhealthy to have sex. In such conditions, a man will not force her and if he does, it's cruelty. We don't regard it as rape as originally suggested, but it can be a ground for separation. But sex will be denied only if you have a good reason, otherwise marriages will break if you have no genuine reason and you refuse sex ... Making it criminal would bring in the Police and that will be going too far (*New Vision* 14/07/2008).

Museveni also attracted the ire of women's groups by questioning publicly the urgency of enacting the proposed legislation. He argued that the Bill was divisive and that it had 'raised a lot of public outcry and it is something which is not urgently needed. I am going to talk to Cabinet and the concerned committee and see if it can be put aside for the time being, and it will be brought back after some consultations' (*New Vision* 20/04/2005). At the time of writing (April 2010) a number of the issues raised by the Bill remain unresolved.

Many Ugandan women are trapped within a rigid gender hierarchy that serves to limit their life choices. Early marriage is a fact of life, with 20 percent of girls marrying before the age of 15; a complete dependency on their usually older spouses is often assured. By the age of 18, nearly 50 percent of women are married. This contrasts dramatically with figures for men, who, on average, marry at 22 years (Ugandan Government 2006). Adultery is illegal, and its definition is far more stringent for women than it is for men. Likewise, the burden of proof in demonstrating spousal adultery is far higher for women (Ssenyonjo 2007). The vulnerability of women is exacerbated by cultural norms that strip them of control of their bodies. For example, in the Pokot and Sabiny communities in eastern Uganda, female genital cutting remains widespread. Despite government condemnation, the practice continues to be legal. In Uganda generally, domestic violence rates are high and widows are routinely deprived of their husband's property, leaving them destitute (HRW 2003).

With regard to gender and HIV/AIDS, the government's strong emphasis on fidelity is in many ways misplaced. Data suggest that young Ugandan women in permanent relationships are actually one of the highest 'at risk' groups. A Ugandan government (2006) survey showed that 60 percent of new HIV infections involved married individuals, supposedly a low-risk group. Statistics further suggest that young married women are more likely to become infected than unmarried women in the same age cohort (15–24 years old). In part, this can be explained by low levels of condom usage – only 1 percent of married women aged 15–49 reported using condoms (Ugandan Government 2006). Additionally, there is a close correlation between condom usage and wealth and education levels; the poorest and least educated people make the least use of condoms. Given that Ugandan women tend to be more disadvantaged in both of these respects than their male counterparts, their ability to make and implement informed decisions regarding sexuality are reduced significantly. Surveys have shown that men are twice as likely as their wives to bring HIV into a relationship (cited in Parikh 2007). Human Rights Watch has documented cases of HIV-infected men, aware of their status, insisting on intercourse without recourse to condoms (HRW 2003). Essentially, if behavioural change truly has been a feature of the Ugandan experience, prevalence rates amongst married couples should be declining; they are not.

Conclusion

Uganda is lodged firmly in the global mindset as an African HIV/AIDS success story and, given the unrelentingly depressing news associated with the pandemic, it is only natural for a success story to be celebrated widely. It is also only natural that the 'Ugandan model' should have engendered plans for duplication in other African countries. Defining this model is, however, problematic. Some have argued that there is no model to replicate and that the extent of the 'miracle' has either been exaggerated by those with vested interests or that the data can be explained away without reference to policy interventions. However, what has truly divided AIDS campaigners is the prioritization, by senior government officials and FBOs, of a morality-centred approach to combating the disease, derided by critics as an 'Anything But Condoms' perspective. The extent to which the religious convictions of FBOs and influential individuals should determine policy measures like condom distribution is hugely problematic for secular activists. Given the scope and influence of FBOs like the Catholic Church in sub-Saharan Africa, particularly in their funding and treatment of HIV/AIDS, religiously-motivated actors must be offered due consideration. That being said, the moral framework being advocated is one that reinforces gender hierarchies and, as a result, young women are arguably being put at greater risk of exposure to HIV, even if they adhere to the basic tenets of the 'social vaccine's' behavioural change message.

8
Governance, the International Trading System and Access to Antiretrovirals

The question of universal access to life-saving drugs like antiretrovirals is inevitably emotive. ARVs are the only proven means of staving off AIDS. That so many in Africa do not have access to ARVs is clearly problematic, both morally and medically. The need for a comprehensive biomedical framework for African states has never been more urgent. An obvious starting point for consideration is cost. Here, the HIV/AIDS story comes with a ready made villain in the shape of the multinational pharmaceutical giants, perceived by some critics to be making billions of dollars in profits whilst people across sub-Saharan Africa die. Campaigners pressing for universal access to ARVs point to the influence of 'Big Pharma' in driving and shaping both American and WTO policies on the protection of intellectual property rights with respect to the patenting of their products. The extension of these rights across the globe has cemented the major drug companies' control over the international pharmaceutical market and, with it, their ability to control prices and access. The rules regulating the governance of international trade are thus pivotal to the future of HIV/AIDS treatment, particularly in poorer countries where price concerns can mean the difference between life and death.

The role of multinational pharmaceutical companies in HIV/AIDS management has become controversial largely due to the increased protection afforded to the intellectual property rights of their products. The vehicle for this has been the 1994 Trade Related Aspects of Intellectual Property Rights (TRIPS) agreement. TRIPS forms part of the WTO framework – and was something for which the US government campaigned strenuously during the Uruguay Round negotiations (1986 to 1994) that culminated in the creation in 1995, as a successor to GATT,[1] of the WTO itself. The TRIPS regulations, along with the 'TRIPS-plus' elements inherent in American bilateral free trade agreements, have been viewed as attempts by the mainly American pharmaceutical giants to limit access to drugs and to ration resources based on an ability to pay. The drug companies' main argument in defence of what they themselves agree are substantial profits is that profits drive research and development. Given the excessive costs, both in terms of time and capital outlay inherent in the development of new drugs, without recompense innovation would cease. Given that a new generation of ARV therapies will be needed in the coming decades as patients build up resistance to existing medicines, such a shift could be potentially catastrophic. Furthermore, without an incentive to invest in the 'diseases of the poor', drug companies could conceivably concentrate on less controversial markets dealing with developed-world conditions including high blood pressure, cholesterol and heart disease, and abandon research into diseases like malaria and tuberculosis. Evidence already suggests that drug companies are increasingly leaving the development of a HIV/AIDS vaccine to bodies sponsored by charitable organizations like the Bill and Melinda Gates Foundation.

Crucially, competition from generic producers operating outwith the parameters of intellectual property rights has cut dramatically the cost of access to first-line therapies, from over $10,000 per year to just $123 per year for some therapies (WHO 2007a). Competition from generic producers is therefore 'obviously' a good thing when it comes to driving down prices. However, drug companies point out that price is just one aspect of the wider HIV/AIDS governance conundrum. They emphasize consideration of the 'bigger picture'. They argue that prices have little to do with access and that ARVs, even at $123 per year, remain outside of the reach of those earning less than $1 per day. They point instead to the crumbling or non-existent sub-Saharan healthcare infrastructure and lack of medical personnel as being far greater barriers to successful treatment. However, despite the significant increases in ARV funding provided by PEPFAR, the Global Fund and the World Bank (Chapter 6), the fact remains that funds are limited and costs do play a part in determining access. The aggressive tactics employed by Big Pharma, in conjunction with the US government, against what it perceives to be the cavalier approach towards intellectual property rights of developing countries including Brazil, India, South Africa and Thailand do little to dispel the caricature of villainous corporations profiting at the expense of the poor. While TRIPS itself offers poorer countries the opportunity to circumvent intellectual property rights, the fact that so few have chosen to do so, despite clear evidence of need, is indicative of the power of Big Pharma and US trade policy. Generic producers are increasingly being brought under the auspices of TRIPS and there is a real fear that new AIDS treatments, so-called second-line therapies, might result in a North-South split in availability, based on price and ability to pay. This means that the fight to drive down drug prices, largely accomplished around 2000, will potentially need to be fought anew.

Big Pharma, profits and the poor

In terms of biomedical treatments, pharmaceutical companies have long been targeted as the villains of the HIV/AIDS story. A highly significant 2001 court case brought against the South African government by 39 multinational pharmaceutical companies over issues of copyright, licensing and the purchasing of HIV/AIDS generic drugs was for those companies an unmitigated public relations disaster that appeared to confirm the primary stereotype associated with Big Pharma; the prioritization of profits over human life. The American-based conglomerates of Pfizer, Johnson & Johnson, Merck & Co, Eli Lilly & Company, Proctor & Gamble, and Bristol-Meyers Sqibb are global household names. Collectively, in 2006, they, and other top ten economic pharmaceutical performers produced profits of nearly $40 billion in an international market worth close $640 billion (Waxman 2006). That these almost obscenely profitable drug companies could band together to try to prevent the distribution of cheap life-saving drugs to some of the poorest and most vulnerable people in the world was viewed with ill-disguised contempt and anger. Big Pharma has also been accused of attempting to influence the outcome of US- and WTO-initiated efforts to tighten the regulations surrounding the manufacturing, distribution and sale of generic drugs.

In the interests of fostering pharmaceutical innovation, research and development, drug company advocates argue that it is vital that intellectual property rights be protected. It is claimed that it costs up to $800 million and takes between ten and 15 years to bring a new drug to market (PhRMA 2007). In 2005 alone, drug companies were said to have spent nearly $40 billion on research and development (GAO 2006). Without financial incentive, the argument goes, innovation will be curtailed and drug companies will focus their energies on 'blockbuster' drugs that treat the conditions of the developed world: cholesterol (Lipitor), blood pressure (Norvasc), depression (Zoloft) and cold sores (Valtrex). 'Third world diseases', already marginalized, will become unprofitable. At the same time, the human cost of high drug prices can be calculated, literally, in terms of millions of lives either lost or at risk. The WHO's (2007a) 'Towards Universal Access' report demonstrates that the number of sub-Saharan African HIV/AIDS sufferers receiving treatment has improved dramatically; the approximately 100,000 people on ARVs (a coverage of 2 percent) at the beginning of 2004 had, by 2007, become 1.34 million (a coverage of 28 percent). The most recent reports from the WHO indicate that this level has now reached 44 percent (WHO 2009g). However, these improved figures also show that universal access remains some way off.

Cost is a critical factor in the rollout of ARVs. 97 percent of the people receiving treatment in low- and middle-income developing countries are receiving first-line ARV therapy. The more sophisticated and less toxic second-line therapies remain prohibitively expensive (WHO 2008a). While costs have fallen dramatically in the past decade, with the most commonly used first-line fixed-dose combination (stavudine + lamivudine + nevirapine) now costing just US$123 per person per year (WHO 2007a), this figure remains well beyond the reach of those living on less than a dollar a day. Universal access to ARVs requires, amongst other factors, an even more significant price drop and far greater flexibility where intellectual property rights are concerned. However, if apologists for the drug companies are correct in arguing that a lack of financial incentive will stifle innovation, there is a further possibility that this will also lead to the holy grail of a vaccine or cure for HIV/AIDS being left on the backburner. At the same time, it might also be that the debate over costing is a red herring and that drug prices, whilst important, are not the determining factor in deciding universal access – after all, few African countries possess the necessary healthcare infrastructure to facilitate a mass rollout of ARVs, even if the drugs themselves were to be provided free of charge. As the head of HIV/AIDS at the WHO, Dr Kevin De Cock, has put it, 'if you work in these countries, it is very obvious very quickly that the elephant in the room is not the current prices of drugs. The real obstacle is the fragility of the health systems, particularly in Africa' (cited in Tabe 2006).

Conspiracy-type theories based around Big Pharma are largely one-dimensional and do little to engage with the question of how to ensure universal access. While drug companies have certainly acted provocatively at times, especially during the 1990s, neither they nor TRIPS are at fault for the poor coverage of those in need of treatment. In the same way that famine is rarely caused solely by a lack of food, the lack of access to drugs can only partly be explained by the voraciousness of pharmaceutical multinationals and the inequitable system of global trade.

Drug prices and universal access to ARVs

The efficacy of ARVs, together with other HIV/AIDS treatments like Cotrimoxazole prophylaxis, a treatment for HIV/AIDS sufferers also battling tuberculosis, has been notable. Without treatment, the life expectancy for someone with HIV is approximately 12 years (Hogg 2006). Due to ARVs, since the late 1990s, life expectancy has increased by approximately 13 years (Hogg 2006). Current estimates suggest that a 20-year-old infected with the virus could, in a developed country, expect to live into his/her fifties. Accordingly, in many developed countries HIV/AIDS is now perceived to be a 'manageable' disease rather a death sentence. Since 2002, the rollout of ARVs in low- and middle-income countries has resulted in approximately three million people being treated with ARVs, over two million of whom live in sub-Saharan Africa (WHO 2008a). Similarly, research suggests that ARVs, in combination with other drugs, can cut mortality rates by 95 percent. It is thus clear that, with ready access to first-line therapies alone, the lives of literally millions in sub-Saharan Africa could be extended significantly.

The practicalities inherent in offering treatment to literally tens of millions of people are undoubtedly complex. Universal access to care is unquestionably a noble goal, but progressing beyond liberal sentiment requires coordination and cooperation between multiple actors on an extraordinary scale. In 2001, the UN General Assembly adopted the Declaration of Commitment on HIV/AIDS in which it established a number of goals and priorities for combating the pandemic. The Declaration emphasized the importance of both the drug companies and the international trading system in ensuring the widest possible availability of access to treatment. The wording made it clear that the international regime governing trade, especially with respect to the protection of intellectual property rights, should not to be allowed to operate as an obstacle to universal access to medication. The TRIPS regime, it was noted, contained a number of 'loopholes' allowing countries to take steps to protect citizens in the case of healthcare emergencies. UN member states were therefore encouraged, by the declaration, while working within the stated rules of the WTO to build up their domestic capacities in order to facilitate access to necessary medicines, including, potentially, the development of a generic pharmaceutical capacity. The Declaration expressly welcomed:

> the efforts of countries to promote innovation and the development of domestic industries consistent with international law in order to

increase access to medicines to protect the health of their populations ... noting that the impact of international trade agreements on access to or local manufacturing of essential drugs and on the development of new drugs needs to be evaluated further (UN 2001).

In a follow-up meeting in 2006, the member states of the United Nations reiterated the need for universal access and agreed:

> to [the pursuit of] all necessary efforts to scale up nationally driven, sustainable and comprehensive responses to achieve broad multi-sectoral coverage for prevention, treatment, care and support, with full and active participation of people living with HIV, vulnerable groups, most affected communities, civil society and the private sector, towards the goal of universal access to comprehensive prevention programmes, treatment, care and support [and we] recognize further that to mount a comprehensive response, we must overcome any legal, regulatory, trade and other barriers that block access to prevention, treatment, care and support (UN 2006a).

As of 2010, the target of universal access has by no means been reached. At the same time, access has improved significantly since 2000. In the 'Towards Universal Access' report, the WHO (2007a) put the number of people in need of antiretroviral therapy in sub-Saharan Africa at nearly five million, of whom 1.34 million were receiving treatment. By 2008, this figure had increased to 2.12 million (WHO 2008a).

In terms of coverage, this increase represents only a marginal improvement, because between 2007 and 2008, the number of people requiring treatment rose from five to seven million. Nonetheless, there have been dramatic improvements in ensuring access for those affected and it is clear that this increase in coverage has been, at least in part, facil-itated by a dramatic fall in the prices of first-line ARVs. The WHO's (2009b) Global Price Reporting Mechanism demonstrates that in low-income countries, between 2003 and 2006, ARV prices fell between 37 and 53 percent, depending on the nature of the regimen. In middle-income countries, the fall, while not as dramatic, still averaged between 10 and 20 percent over the same period. Based on these raw figures, it would suggest that there is a direct correlation between falling prices and improved access to treatment. If so, then the case against the avarice of multinational drug companies is compelling and unequivocal.

Table 8.1   ARV Coverage by Country

Country	Percentage of HIV+ Persons Receiving Antiretroviral Therapy 2004	Percentage of HIV+ Persons Receiving Antiretroviral Therapy 2007
Angola	9	25
Benin	13	49
Botswana	44	79
Cameroon	9	25
Central African Republic	3	21
Congo, Republic of the	2	17
Côte d'Ivoire	3	28
Democratic Republic of the Congo	4	24
Djibouti	6	16
Equatorial Guinea	<1	31
Eritrea	<1	13
Ethiopia	4	29
Ghana	3	15
Kenya	6	38
Lesotho	4	26
Malawi	5	35
Mozambique	3	24
Namibia	22	88
Nigeria	2	26
Rwanda	10	71
Senegal	26	56
South Africa	4	28
Swaziland	14	42
Uganda	12	33
Zambia	7	46
Zimbabwe	1	18

Source: (UNAIDS 2008d)

Protecting intellectual property rights

Particularly with respect to pharmaceuticals, TRIPS has created a storm of controversy ever since its inception in 1994. The dramatic escalation of the African HIV/AIDS crisis during the course of the 1990s has made it more controversial still. At the heart of concerns over the potential human cost of TRIPS is a fear that multinational pharmaceutical companies have hijacked the international trading regime, imposing their concept of 'order' on what had previously been a somewhat anarchical international system.

The TRIPS agreement covers elements like copyright and rights related to copyright and industrial property. The agreement obliges member states to offer a predetermined minimum level of protection for patents and trademarks, and ensures that individual patents remain protected for a period of 20 years (Brant 2003). Prior to TRIPS, patent protection generally lasted 15–17 years in developed countries and approximately 5–7 years in developing countries (WHO 2005). TRIPS created a global standard for patent protection where, in the past, none had existed. International patent protection dates back to the Paris Convention for the Protection of Industrial Property in 1883. It has been periodically updated and renewed ever since, but it has never stipulated minimum standards of patent protection amongst its signatory states (Ryan 1998).

The original catalyst for the 1883 Convention was the need to prevent national governments from discriminating against foreign patent holders. The 1883 treaty also made provision for compulsory licensing in order to prevent 'abuses' arising from the exercising of patents.[2] A number of additional treaties followed: the Berne Convention for the Protection of Literary and Artistic Works (1886), the Madrid Agreement Concerning the International Registration of Marks (1891), the Hague Agreement Concerning the International Registration of Industrial Designs (1925), the Rome Convention for the Protection of Performers, Producers of Phonograms and Broadcasting Organizations (1961), the Patent Cooperation Treaty (1970), the Geneva Convention for the Protection of Producers of Phonograms Against Unauthorized Duplication of their Phonograms (1971), the Budapest Treaty on the International Recognition of the Deposit of Micro-organisms for the Purposes of Patent Procedure (1977).

TRIPS differs from the these forerunners in that, unlike the majority of international agreements, it is based not on the lowest common denominator, but the highest; the global trading system was, after the inception of TRIPS, almost at a stroke forced to comply with First World intellectual property rules. Prior to TRIPS, a number of developing countries either did not have laws protecting intellectual property with respect to medicines or simply offered protection for production processes rather than actual products. India, for example, one of the world's largest producers of generic drugs, did not, prior to 1995, offer patents for products *per se*. It provided patents for the processes developed to manufacture them. Brazil, another major producer of generic drugs, only began to offer patents for pharmaceuticals in 1997. Prior to TRIPS, it was therefore ostensibly permissible for drug companies in India and Brazil to reproduce drugs patented in the West, provided that the method of manufacture did not mirror the original process. Recognizing the pervasiveness of such 'flexible' legislation, TRIPS afforded developing countries a ten-year window, ending in 2005, in which to affect necessary reforms. (This period was extended for Least Developed Countries until 2016 in order to allow for an extended period of adjustment). The net result of TRIPS, then, is that eventually all member states will have to offer protection for patents filed after 1995. Significantly, unlike most international legislation, TRIPS is, *via* the mechanisms of the WTO, enforceable. Correspondingly, countries found to be in breach of TRIPS regulations can be pursued through the WTO's dispute procedure where the burden of proof lies overwhelmingly with the accused party.

Big Pharma's role in shaping TRIPS

It is important to note the role of Big Pharma in shaping the US government's outlook on intellectual property rights. Between 1998 and 2005, the pharmaceutical industry spent more than $800 million on political lobbying, placing it second only to the insurance industry in its attempts to shape public policy (Ismail 2005). In 2007, for instance, the Pharmaceutical Research and Manufacturers of America spent $22,733,400 in lobbying the US Congress and various federal agencies, while Pfizer alone spent $13,800,000 (Conlan 2008). Such figures are comparable with those offered by oil (Exxon-Mobil – $16,940,000) and auto interests (General Motors – $14,560,000; Alliance of Automobile Manufacturers – $12,835,527). It is hardly surprising, given this degree of funding, that the interests of the pharmaceutical sector are taken seriously on Capitol Hill. However, an analysis of the negotiation process that eventually resulted in TRIPS suggests that this sector was not simply 'influential' in determining the US position; it actively shaped policy on the matter.

For many analysts, the biggest surprise about the pharmaceuticals-applicable elements of TRIPS was that these aspects of the treaty were ever agreed upon at all. TRIPS offers a level of protection for intellectual property that benefits only a relatively small number of developed countries (Tyfield 2008). Given that more than 80 percent of pharmaceutical research and development takes place in developed countries, this was arguably a predictable outcome of the TRIPS negotiations. However, it reduces significantly the Treaty's value to other WTO member states (Balasubramaniam 2002). From the perspective of Big Pharma, the benefits of TRIPS are clear. The pharmaceutical industry has been described as being almost uniquely dependent on patents due to the fact that many drugs are relatively simple to reverse-engineer (Tyfield 2008). This makes the industry particularly susceptible to 'free-riders' and thus, arguably, in need of protection. However, in reality, the threat posed to Big Pharma's profits by the potential loss of market-share in developing countries is negligible, given that 91 percent of Big Pharma's sales take place within developed country markets (Tyfield 2008). The arguments presented in favour of TRIPS by the drug companies during multilateral negotiations were thus largely spurious – it was clear, even prior to TRIPS, that the lack of patent protection in regions like sub-Saharan Africa would barely dent the profitability of the major pharmaceutical companies. Why then, despite such obviously problematic arguments, was Big Pharma able to impose its agenda on the Uruguay Round negotiations that resulted in TRIPS? Similarly, why did India and Brazil, both of which had representation at the negotiations, not fight their corners more effectively? After all, in the build up to the Uruguay Round negotiations, India was bullish in its demand that developing countries be able to exclude pharmaceutical goods from patent protection (Ryan 1998). The answer is that opposition to increased protection for intellectual property rights was effectively nullified in advance of the final negotiations by aggressive US tactics.

In response to opposition from developing countries including India and Brazil, the US worked hard to isolate TRIPS rebels and proved extremely effective in mobilizing the support of the other developed countries during the closed door 'Green Room' negotiations that preceded the agreement. The US also made judicious use of bilateral agreements as a means of smoothing the path of the TRIPS agreement through the negotiations. For 'rebellious' countries – India and Brazil in particular – the US made regular use of Section 301 of the Trade Act of 1974 which allows for the United States Trade Representative (USTR) to take action against countries perceived to be acting in a manner that is unfair or discriminatory to US interests (Puckett and Reynolds 1996). In 1987, the USTR, under pressure from the Pharmaceutical Manufacturers Association (PMA) duly instigated an investigation into Brazil's record on the protection of pharmaceutical patents (Drahos 2002). Brazil's initial intransigence led to a 100 percent retaliatory tariff on Brazilian exports of pharmaceuticals, paper and consumer products to the US (Sell 1995). High-level representations from Brazil and the US met five times between May 1993 and February 1994 in order to hammer out an agreement on patents (Sell 1995). Faced with punitive sanctions, the Brazilian government caved in to US demands and brought about changes in its legislation. The US duly revoked the punitive trade tariffs. The result was that Brazil became increasingly less vocal on the matter of patents. Similarly, in 1991, the USTR launched a Section 301 investigation into India's laws on patent protection. Retaliatory tariffs were not levied because the Indian government agreed, under pressure, to an economic reform package that promised greater protection for patent holders. The upshot was that, during the course of the TRIPS negotiations, opposition to US pharmaceutical interests was either bought off with trade deals or compelled to fall into line as a result of strong-arm tactics. Thus it is that, despite the appearance of consultation and transparency, the negotiated outcome that resulted in TRIPS was rooted in far from democratic circumstances. Revisions made to the Trade Act in 1988 meant that resisting US conditions, even in multilateral forums such as the GATT/WTO, can result in countries being subject to a Section 301 investigation. The ability to impose tough sanctions against those found to be discriminating against US interests invested a significant degree of power in the office of the USTR.

Development NGOs like Oxfam have emphasized how the Industry Functional Advisory Committee on Intellectual Property Rights for Trade Policy Matters (IFAC3), which advises the USTR on matters pertaining to intellectual property, has in the past included representatives from the Pharmaceutical Research and Manufacturers of America (PhRMA), Pfizer and Merck & Co (Brant 2003). In 2005, nine out of the 15 members of the IFAC3 Committee were representatives of the pharmaceutical industry (Mayne 2005). The fingerprints of Big Pharma are evident on documentation emanating from the Committee. A report issued by the IFAC3 in 2004 declared that it is 'essential that traditional tools such as Special 301, the unilateral trade preference programmes and WTO dispute settlement mechanism be aggressively employed to lift levels of intellectual property protection' (cited in Mayne 2005). Similarly, the extensive use of the office of the USTR to secure market dominance is evidenced by the fact that PhRMA lodged 28 complaints with the USTR against developing countries in 2001 and a further 27 in 2002. The majority of these complaints involved compulsory licensing agreements (Mayne 2002b). The culmination of the above is that that the pharmaceutical industry has had, and continues to have, a considerable degree of influence in determining the shape of US demands in matters of trade.

The Big Pharma perspective: Innovation and research and development

The pharmaceutical companies argue that medicines are difficult, time-consuming and expensive to produce – as stated, the often-quoted statistics are that it can cost up to $800 million and between ten and

15 years to get a new medicine to market (PhRMA 2007). PhRMA's website (2010) claims that in 2009 its members invested $45.8 billion in 'discovering and developing new medicines'. The associated costs are high because less than 1 percent of compounds examined at the pre-clinical level graduate to the level of human testing, let alone receive FDA approval (Grabowski 2002). In fact only a fifth of drugs vetted in human trials actually make it to the market. However, drugs are relatively easy and cheap to copy. In the US, generic manufacturers need only to demonstrate bio-equivalency in order to gain approval – a process that can cost as little as one million dollars (Grabowski 2002). The argument is that without patent protection and adequate remuneration drug com-panies will eventually be put off innovation, especially in 'difficult' markets where investment might yield only low returns. In this res-pect, TRIPS performs a necessary function, weighing long-term gains in medical innovation against short-term benefits relating to low costs. The WTO (2008) itself argues that the TRIPS agreement

> is an attempt to narrow the gaps in the way these rights are pro-tected around the world, and to bring them under common inter-national rules. It establishes minimum levels of protection that each government has to give to the intellectual property of fellow WTO members. In doing so, it strikes a balance between the long term benefits and possible short term costs to society. Society benefits in the long term when intellectual property protection encourages creation and invention.

Henry Grabowski (2002) cites Japan as a good case study in the way in which increased protection for intellectual property rights stimulates innovation. Prior to 1976, Japan had relatively permissive patenting laws with respect to pharmaceuticals. As with India and Brazil, it allowed for the patenting of processes rather than products. The result was that the Japanese pharmaceutical sector was built largely around generic production and showed little evidence of original research or inno-vation. On reforming its patenting laws to include product protection, Japan emerged as a major player in the pharmaceutical sector, taking a lead in research and development activity. Studies also demonstrate a strong correlation between the protection of intellectual property rights and levels of investment in research and development (Grabowski 2002). Simply put, countries that incentivize firms to invest time, effort and capital into research and development foster innovation. In a 2006 press release, Miles White (2006), the Chairman and CEO of Abbott Laboratories, a major producer of the first-line protease inhibitor medication that is part of HIV/AIDS treatment, described his company's ongoing battle with the Brazilian government:

> Generic manufacturers have an important role to play in lowering the cost of treatment over time, which offers value to society. But society cannot save its way to health with old treatments that gradually lose their effectiveness and offer no help against new diseases. By definition, generic manufacturers make nothing new. And AIDS is a disease that is always new – due to the constant evolution of the virus – and requires new solutions. Where will these come from if we hobble the patent system that drives innovation?

Thus, from this perspective, while low cost generics may be useful in the short term, their long-term usage risks undermining the possibility of a future cure for HIV/AIDS. There is evidence to suggest that approximately 65 percent of new drugs entering the market would not have done so in the absence of patent protection (Thomas 2001). In 1990, the Commission on Health Research for Development (1990) highlighted the extensive social benefits to be gained from investing in research into 'diseases of the poor'. The argument is that there is little enough incentive for drug companies to invest in 'Third World diseases' as it is, given the limited returns offered by the relevant markets. Without patent protection, there would be no incentive at all.

There is a real concern regarding the lack of research into so-called neglected diseases. Only 1.3 percent of all drugs developed between 1975 and 2004 targeted diseases such as African trypanosomiasis, Chagas disease, helminthiasis, leishmaniasis, malaria, onchocerciasis, and schistosomiasis, all of which affect mainly developing countries (Richards 2006, *New Scientist* 30/09/2006). Only four tropical disease treatments were marketed between 1999 and 2004 (Chirac and Torreele 2006). For the pharmaceutical companies, the numbers are stark; while three-quarters of the world's population live in developing countries, they account for just a tenth of global sales in pharmaceuticals (Mayne 2002a). The fact that per capita spending on health in the Africa region of the WHO (2009e) is just $27 as opposed to $1,350 in Europe is indicative of the lack of markets. With respect to HIV/AIDS, the trend is no less discouraging. Evidence from the Global Forum for Health Research (2006) shows a decline between 2002 and 2004 in internally-generated commercial sector funding for research and development into a vaccine against HIV. Much of the research and development funding in this area is now derived from public funds or the philanthropic sector; in 2005, the Bill and Melinda Gates Foundation pledged $360 million towards funding for research into a HIV vaccine (Global Forum for Health Research 2006).

Arguments in favour of protective patenting have, therefore, a certain grim economic rationale, but the foundations on which they are built remain somewhat flimsy. Throughout the pharmaceutical industry in general, innovation is in short supply. The majority of medicines patented are simply modified versions of established products (Correa 2007). A 2002 report by the National Institute for Health Care Management (2002) assessed the levels of innovation inherent in all branded drugs to come onto the market between 1989 and 2000. During this period, the FDA approved 1,035 new drug applications. Of these, only 35 percent were effectively new molecular entities (NMES) or, simply put, truly new drugs. Of the remainder, 65 percent contained active ingredients that were already available for purchase and only differed from their predecessors in terms of either dosage, administration or their combination with other active ingredients. Such 'incrementally modified' formulas thus formed the bulk of new medicines produced. The remaining 11 percent of approvals were for drugs that were identical to existing products (National Institute for Health Care Management 2002). Of the incrementally modified formulas, only 24 percent were deemed to offer a 'significant clinical improvement' over products already on the market. The FDA ruled that, even in the case of the new molecular entities, 58 percent offered little improvement on those which were already commercially available; only 15 percent were deemed to be 'priority-rated' (National Institute for Health Care Management 2002). Furthermore, it is possible to argue that not only are 'innovation' claims by the pharmaceutical industry overstated, but that the development of a pharmaceutical 'anti-commons' might in fact stifle innovation (Sampath 2005). Innovative products and procedures are rarely cut from whole cloth and, by offering a broad platform for patents on medicines, there is a concern that potential advances 'downstream' will be curtailed heavily. After all, most 'innovation' is a collective process, with researchers, to quote Sir Isaac Newton, 'standing on the shoulders of giants' (cited in Hilborn and Liermann 1998). Moreover, the main driving force behind innovation is arguably the 'first mover' principle, in which, as a result of brand recognition, the innovator dominates the market long after competitors enter the arena (Picciotto 2002).

The undeniably contentious nature of TRIPS generated accusations – particularly in the early days of the agreement – that the drug companies had 'captured' the WTO agenda with the aim of creating a 'First

World cartel' controlling global drug production and distribution. There was a fear that generic drug companies would be driven out of business and that key drugs would be priced outside the reach of the poor. HIV/AIDS campaigners, particularly around the time that the Doha negotiations began in 2001, were particularly concerned with the shape of the international trading system, given that they had witnessed generic drug companies slash the price of HIV/AIDS treatment from approximately $10,000 per year in the mid-1990s to a fraction of that barely half a decade later (Brant 2003; WHO 2007a). In this respect, Big Pharma has not aided its cause. For all their talk of research and development costs, the fact is that the major pharmaceutical companies are almost obscenely profitable. Their aggressive lobbying tactics and obstructionist interventions such as those involving the USTR, have done little to quell the fears of critics sceptical of their motives.

Making use of loopholes: TRIPS and compulsory licensing

On paper, TRIPS does not represent a 'blank cheque' for pharmaceutical companies. The agreement, while loaded in favour of the drug companies, takes into account the special nature of pharmaceuticals, acknowledging that drugs cannot be conceived of in quite the same manner as CDs or DVDs. The actual TRIPS agreement is relatively flexible, allowing governments to sanction the use of patents without the concurrence of patent holders if the need arises. Specifically, TRIPS makes provision for national emergencies – situations in which health concerns supersede intellectual property protection. Such public health safeguards are covered by articles 6, 8, 30 and 31 of the agreement. Article 31 states that patents can be overridden 'in the case of a national emergency or other circumstances of extreme urgency' (WTO 1994). Under Article 31, governments can issue compulsory licences allowing for the production of any drugs without patent holders' permission, provided 'adequate' compensation is paid. Parallel importing, whereby governments can authorize the import of drugs purchasable abroad for less than the cost of domestically-produced medicines, is also sanctioned, providing – and this is the critical point – such an option forms part of the exporter's national legislation (drug prices vary dramatically from country to country, usually determined by the drug companies on the basis of perceived ability to pay).

Although TRIPS allows for a degree of 'flexibility' with respect to medicines, the rules for circumventing patent protection are nonetheless onerous for developing countries. As a result, instances of 'national emergency' relating to health are seldom invoked. Where governments have attempted to import cheaper generic medicines, their efforts have been resisted stoutly by the drug companies holding the patents. Glaxo-SmithKline, for example, has fought attempts by Ghana and Uganda to import generic versions of its ARV Combivir. However, the case that caused the greatest degree of controversy, and put the motives of the pharmaceutical industry under the spotlight, was the 1997 attempt by 39 pharmaceutical companies, including GlaxoSmithKline, to take the South African government to court over its Medicines and Related Substances Act.

The aim of the Medicines and Related Substances Act was to alter the South African patent regime in the interests of legalizing the import of generic HIV/AIDS drugs from producers including India and Brazil (Sidley 2001). At stake was amendment 15(c) of the Act which allows for TRIPS-compliant compulsory licensing and the parallel importation of pharmaceuticals. The case against South Africa, originally filed in February 1998, came to trial in March 2001 amidst unprecedented publicity. However, before it could unfold fully, the pharmaceutical companies withdrew their suit, a move lamented by interested parties like the Treatment Action Campaign, which had hoped to see some form of precedent set in favour of developing countries' utilization of the TRIPS flexibilities. The presiding judge himself was at pains to highlight the international importance of the case (Mayne 2002a). Universal access campaigners had hoped that a legal ruling against the drug companies would encourage other developing countries to be bold in their use of compulsory licensing and parallel importing. The irony was, of course, that, having successfully resisted the combined might of the drug companies, the South African government did little to ensure further the right of universal access for AIDS sufferers, with the result being the 2007 access rate of just 28 percent (see Table 8.1).

The aggressive actions of the pharmaceutical companies towards South Africa prompted developing countries to press for a review of the TRIPS regime as part of the WTO Doha Round negotiations, launched in 2001 (negotiations that are yet to be finalized despite having been scheduled for completion in 2005). Pressure from member states led to the enactment of the Doha Declaration on the TRIPS Agreement and Public Health in November 2001, which spelt out the primacy of access over patent rights:

> We agree that the TRIPS Agreement does not and should not prevent Members from taking measures to protect public health. Accordingly,

while reiterating our commitment to the TRIPS Agreement, we affirm that the Agreement can and should be interpreted and implemented in a manner supportive of WTO Members' right to protect public health and, in particular, to promote access to medicines for all (WTO 2001 – Paragraph 4).

The 2001 Declaration also made provision for poorer countries to circumvent restrictions on their ability to issue compulsory licences:

We recognize that WTO Members with insufficient or no manufacturing capacities in the pharmaceutical sector could face difficulties in making effective use of compulsory licensing under the TRIPS Agreement. We instruct the Council for TRIPS to find an expeditious solution to this problem (WTO 2001 – Paragraph 6).

However, despite these early encouraging signs that TRIPS was being shaped to prioritize the needs of the sick in regions like Africa, this element of the Doha Round has floundered alongside the broader negotiations themselves, largely because there appears to be little enthusiasm for the declaration on the part of the developed countries.

For all the talk of loopholes and flexibilities available to developing countries within the TRIPS Agreement, what is sometimes forgotten, particularly given the strong-arm tactics employed by countries including the US with respect to the enforcement of patent rights, is that many developed countries, including the US, Australia, Canada, Germany, Ireland, Italy and the United Kingdom, have themselves been happy to bend the rules where the issuing of compulsory licences is concerned. For example, the US government, under legislation covered by 28 United States Code s. 1498, is able to ride roughshod over patent laws in the interests of the public good (Love 2002). Canada, prior to joining NAFTA in 2000, regularly issued compulsory licences for drugs.

Compulsory licensing does not represent a complete loss for patent holders. TRIPS provides some protection for the drug companies in this regard, ensuring that royalties are paid to relevant parties. Article 31 (h) of the TRIPS Agreement states that 'the right holder shall be paid adequate remuneration in the circumstances of each case, taking into account the economic value of the authorisation'. The reality, however, is that TRIPS allows states to be reasonably flexible in determining the degree of compensation afforded to patent holders, with the result being that patent holders and compulsory-licence issuers differ as to what constitutes an adequate level of compensation. PhRMA, representing companies including Bayer, GlaxoSmithKline and Johnson & Johnson, has argued in favour of a 5 percent royalty rate. In practice, royalties can vary, with Japan, for instance, historically offering rates of between 2 and 4 percent, Germany between 2 and 10 percent and Canada an average of 4 percent (Love 2002).

Big Pharma's role in shaping the US TRIPS-plus agenda

The stalled status of the Doha Round negotiations notwithstanding, by the end of the Seattle Ministerial Conference in 1999 it was clear that the developed countries had lost a certain degree of their power to influence the agenda of the WTO. The major pharmaceutical companies, while initially satisfied with the TRIPS agreement as it originally stood in the mid-1990s, became somewhat frustrated with the lengthy compliance periods subsequently awarded to developing countries and Least Developed Countries (until 2005 for developing countries, and until 2016 for LDCs). In addition, especially post-2001, the softening of the language on intellectual property rights with respect to pharmaceuticals meant that Big Pharma became increasingly focused on circumventing WTO flexibilities.

Pharmaceutical interests began to exert increasing pressure on the US government to both employ more aggressively the Section 301 process and conduct bilateral negotiations with developing countries in the interests of ensuring TRIPS compliance ahead of schedule (Drahos 2002). In terms of producing generic HIV/AIDS drugs, this meant that poorer countries that might still have been able to benefit from the TRIPS 'phasing-in' period came under increasing pressure to conform ahead of time to Big Pharma demands. From the late 1990s onwards, the US began to insist that potential partners in bilateral free trade agreements agree to offer a standard of intellectual property protection similar to that offered within the US – so-called TRIPS-plus conditionality. Given that the US is in the process of negotiating a free trade agreement with the Southern African Customs Union (Botswana, Lesotho, Namibia, South Africa and Swaziland – countries that are at the epicentre of the HIV/AIDS pandemic), the ramifications for universal access to ARVs could be potentially significant. As with TRIPS, US free trade agreements call for 20-year patent protection and require that delays in securing market access, such as safety and quality checks, be added to this period. Where pharmaceuticals are concerned, the agreements also constrain partner countries from issuing compulsory licences. Exceptions are emergencies, efforts to overcome antitrust issues, and cases of public non-commercial use (Fink and Reichenmiller 2006). However, the agreements also impose additional restrictions that have significant ramifications for generic producers. Crucially, TRIPS-plus conditions usually insist on the protection of patent-holder test data for five years. This level of data protection means that generic producers cannot simply demonstrate the bio-equivalence of their products. It means that they are also obliged to secure independent data demonstrating the safety and efficacy of their products, which can be both time-consuming and exceptionally expensive (Fink and Reichenmiller 2006). Lastly, as opposed to TRIPS, the US free trade agreements place restrictions on parallel importing. As the WTO has worked towards making TRIPS acceptable to poorer countries, so the US, at the instigation of Big Pharma, has worked towards circumventing concessions. The practice of integrating TRIPS-plus conditionality into its bilateral free trade agreements therefore puts the US at odds with the WTO over its TRIPS provisions that facilitate the protection of public health and 'enhance access to medicines for poor countries' (WTO 2001).

Big Pharma and the US undermine TRIPS flexibilities

The TRIPS-plus provisions outlined above run counter to the spirit of the compromise agreement reached by WTO members in 2003 to allow countries with insufficient industrial capacity to important generic drugs made under compulsory licence (WTO 2003). A great deal of optimism accompanied this agreement, which waived countries' obligations under Article 31 (f) of TRIPS, which states that medicines produced under compulsory licence must be for domestic consumption. The then Director-General of the WTO, Supachai Panitchpakdi, declared the compromise to be

> the final piece of the jigsaw ... allowing poorer countries to make full use of the flexibilities in the WTO's intellectual property rules in order to deal with the diseases that ravage their people. It proves once and for all that the organization can handle humanitarian as well as trade concerns' (WTO 2003).

However, the flexibilities inherent in TRIPS have not delivered results on the ground. Rwanda is the only country to have taken the opportunity to import generic drugs made under compulsory licence (Kategekwa 2009). Thailand, lauded in development circles for its public health policies, has at the urging of Big Pharma come under sustained pressure to acquiesce to TRIPS-plus restrictions (Kripke and Weinberg 2006). The role of the US and Big Pharma in blocking the Thai government's attempts to provide cheap HIV/AIDS medicines is illustrative of the determination of the pharmaceutical sector to undermine the ability of poorer countries to exploit the flexibilities afforded by TRIPS. In response to the HIV/AIDS pandemic, the Thai government successfully established a generic pharmaceutical sector and, by 2002, was offering domestically-produced ARVs at a fraction of the cost of their branded counterparts. Some of these medicines, such as the Abbott-owned ARV Kaletra, were produced under compulsory licence. The net result of the burgeoning domestic drug-producing sector was an eight-fold expansion in Thailand's rollout of ARVs (Kripke and Weinberg 2006). In response to this public health triumph, the major drug companies have pursued action against the Thai government through both the courts and bilateral trade negotiations. Despite political hurdles such as the overthrow of Thai Prime Minister Thaksin Shinawatra in 2006, and the resulting suspension of formal free trade agreement[3] negotiations, high-level bilateral trade talks between the two countries have continued, with the USTR applying pressure on Thailand to accede to a TRIPS-plus framework in exchange for greater access to US markets.

The US has employed similar tactics against Brazil. Brazil has been most successful in delivering access to ARVs, with near-universal coverage being achieved by 2006 (Steinbrook 2007). In May 2007, after its negotiations with the company broke down, the Brazilian government issued compulsory licences for Efavirenz, a Merck & Co product. In response, a Merck spokesperson complained that measures of this nature amounted to an undermining of intellectual property rights that might well jeopardize future medical innovation:

> Research and development-based pharmaceutical companies like Merck simply cannot sustain a situation in which the developed countries alone are expected to bear the cost for essential drugs in both least-developed countries and emerging markets. As such, we believe it is essential to price our medicines according to a country's level of development and HIV burden, thereby ensuring equitable access as well as our ability to invest in future innovative medicines (Alcorn 2007).

After being lobbied by the pharmaceutical sector, the USTR went on to place Brazil on its 'watch list' due to what the former referred to as a 'proliferation' of the manufacturing of 'counterfeit' pharmaceuticals. In light of its lobbying and influence over the USTR, it is reasonable to accuse Big Pharma of attempting to limit access to its products by virtue of trade practices that ensure an oligarchic closed shop. In seeking to prevent or curtail competition from generic manufacturers, Big Pharma's actions can be viewed as attempts (intentional or not) to ration access to medicine (Sell 2007). Arguably, other countries have not followed Thailand's lead in developing generic medicine sectors because the potential economic costs and tradeoffs of offending US pharmaceutical interests are simply too high.

At the same time, it is also arguable that evidence of companies 'profiteering' from the sale of HIV/AIDS medication in Africa has been exaggerated greatly. Particularly in the aftermath of the South African court debacle, many drug companies, including Merek & Co, Bristol-Meyers Squibb and GlaxoSmithKline, slashed the prices of their AIDS-fighting drugs and worked hard to rehabilitate their battered images. In July 2009, GlaxoSmithKilne (2009b) announced that it had granted South African generics producer Aspen permission to produce Abacavir as part of a royalty-free voluntary licence. In order to bolster research into tropical diseases, the company also offered to place a number of its patents for so-called neglected diseases in a 'patent-pool' (Glaxo-SmithKilne 2009a). Similarly, in August 2009, Pfizer entered into an agreement with the Clinton Foundation (2009) to cut the cost of Rifa-butin, its TB treatment for HIV sufferers, by 60 percent. The deal will see Pfizer undercutting rival generic producers in China and India.

However, even if drug companies were to be found to be keeping drug prices high, the effect of pricing on access to medicine in sub-Saharan Africa remains open to question. In 2005, global expenditure on health-care equated to I\$5.1 trillion,[4] but this average belies a number of extremes. Across much of the African continent, healthcare spending equates to less than US\$10 per capita, with the Democratic Republic of Congo (DRC) spending just US\$0.50 per citizen (WHO 2008c). For citizens of countries like the DRC, HIV/AIDS medication, generic or otherwise, is simply beyond reach.

The accessibility of second-line therapies

At the individual level, then, it would seem that the price of drugs may be largely irrelevant where the treatment of HIV/AIDS across much of sub-Saharan Africa is concerned. Nearly half of the people living in the region subsist on less than a dollar per day, thereby discounting them as paying consumers of any drugs, generic or otherwise (World Bank 2007). Drug companies have correctly emphasized how cost is not the key factor in preventing universal access, and that, even if ARVs were free, the infrastructure necessary to administer universal healthcare programmes for sufferers does not exist in some countries (Chapter 5).

Still, as suggested above, the gap between developed and developing countries with respect to HIV/AIDS treatment is epitomized by levels of access to second-line treatments. Over time, patients on first-line therapies can build up resistance to these regimes, which nullifies their efficacy. While there are generic equivalents for most first-line therapies, the same is not true for their second-line counterparts, with the newer drugs currently eight to 12 times more expensive (MSF 2009). What separates first-line from second-line therapies in terms of patent protection is that the majority of second-line therapies were patented after countries like India and Brazil amended their patenting laws and became TRIPS-compliant. Consequently, these drugs are afforded far greater levels of protection than drugs patented in the early 1990s. Under Indian law, drugs patented after 1 January 1995 are afforded full TRIPS consideration. Medicines pioneered prior to this date are not offered the same protection. The result is that India, despite having a sophisticated generic industry, has no plans to incorporate a mass rollout of second-line ARVs under the government's free treatment programme (Alliance India 2006). Only 2 percent of those receiving treatment for HIV/AIDS in low- and middle-income countries are receiving second-line therapy (WHO 2007b).

In sub-Saharan Africa, 96 percent of drug procurement is spent on first-line therapy, with just 4 percent going to second-line treatments (Chien 2007). Of the first-line therapies, 65 percent are sourced from generic manufacturers while with respect to second-line drugs this figure falls to just 7 percent (Chien 2007). While generic first-line drugs were significantly cheaper, generic second-line treatments are no cheaper than branded versions (Chien 2007). As increasing numbers of people come to receive first-line therapies, so the number of cases of resistance and toxicity will necessitate an eventual shift to second-line therapies. The WHO (2007b) estimates a shift of 3 percent per year. However, if prices for second-line therapies do not begin to fall dramatically, public health programmes could conceivably end up allocating as much as 90 percent of their therapy budgets to such medications (WHO 2007b).

Part of the problem for generic companies wanting to expand into the HIV/AIDS sector is the shift towards data protection. In countries tied to free trade agreements with the US, this safety and efficacy data is off-limits to competitors for up to five years. While compulsory licensing remains an option under TRIPS, and countries like Mozambique, Zambia and Zimbabwe have all issued compulsory licences for first-line therapies, most countries have been reluctant to make use of this option. Given the examples of Thailand and Brazil, as outlined above, this is hardly surprising. Only by virtue of being the world's 12th largest economy has Brazil been prepared to take on the pharmaceutical giants over first-line therapies. It has been less bold in developing its capacity to produce second-line drugs. It is thus clear that, although compulsory licensing exists as an option in theory, very few countries feel sufficiently confident to defy the US or Big Pharma in exercising their rights with regard to second-line therapies. Moreover, drug companies such as Abbott are now actively withholding the registration of drugs in certain countries until the respective governments agree in advance to forego compulsory licensing (MSF 2007). With respect to second-line treatments, therefore, there is a pervading sense of *déjà vu* very reminiscent of the Big Pharma/South Africa court case of 2001.

Conclusion

Every story needs its villains, and, with respect to HIV/AIDS, Big Pharma, the US government and the WTO represent the most obvious hate-figures. The perception that this is a tale involving greedy multi-billion dollar corporations manipulating governments and international organizations in the interests of profiting from the misery and suffering of some of the poorest people in the world is difficult to escape. At the same time, TRIPS, on paper, is far more flexible than many critics would allow, offering a number of 'emergency clauses', including the right to issue compulsory licences, to governments faced with overwhelming health concerns. The fact that so few countries have invoked these clauses is arguably of more interest than the perceived iniquities of TRIPS itself. In the wake of the stalling of the WTO Doha Round negotiations, the US has embarked on a plethora of bilateral trade initiatives incorporating TRIPS-plus conditionality. In this, the effects of political lobbying by Big Pharma on the US government are evident. The drug companies argue that patent protection is ultimately a positive-sum game because, without safeguards, innovation, research and development would falter. From this perspective, generic companies offer little that is 'value-added' and, ultimately, could stand in the way of future medical breakthroughs. Yet the fact remains that, as competition from generic drug suppliers has increased, so the prices of HIV/AIDS drugs have fallen. Similarly, as prices have fallen, so coverage has increased. On a very basic level, it seems clear that cost and accessibility appear strongly linked. In particular, debates linked to second-line ARVs have highlighted the matter of pricing in prolonging the lives of sufferers who can no longer be treated with first-line therapies.

However, it can be argued that the whole cost debate is a red herring, that even if drugs were free, that millions of AIDS sufferers in Africa would still be without treatment due to insufficient healthcare infrastructure and personnel. The majority of African sufferers do not actually pay for their treatment; they receive it free of charge *via* either national programmes or aid initiatives such as PEPFAR, Global Fund and MAP. This argument is disingenuous for two reasons. Firstly, PEPFAR and Global Fund have limited budgets and costs must be prioritized. Secondly, simply because healthcare infrastructure in sub-Saharan Africa is limited does not imply that cost does not play a role in affecting people's access to medicine; cost is always a contributing factor. It is important, therefore, that the Doha negotiations be re-invigorated and an agreement concluded, because there is potential within the WTO framework for developing countries to make better use of their rights under TRIPS to issue compulsory licences and/or engage in parallel importing. The TRIPS-plus bilateral trade agreements between the US and various developing countries, symptomatic of the failure of the Doha agenda, have merely cemented – and will continue to cement – the international influence of Big Pharma, and to restrict the ability of national governments to act in the interests of their own citizens.

Conclusion

As 'ground zero' for HIV/AIDS, sub-Saharan African has borne the brunt of the pandemic. However, simply explaining HIV/AIDS in sub-Saharan Africa as the latest in a long list of disasters to befall the continent offers little by way of a solution to the crisis. In the same way that a famine is rarely an 'act of God', the extent of the HIV/AIDS pandemic was by no means preordained and can, in some respects at least, be read as a failure of politics and governance at the national, regional and international level. The African AIDS crisis reveals itself as a complexity of interrelated actors, institutions and practices lacking both clearly identifiable 'villains' and simple solutions. The discovery of an effective vaccine or cure would bring true closure to the AIDS crisis. However, in the immediate future at least, the prospects for this are low. For many years to come, it is likely that governance will continue to determine the course of the HIV/AIDS pandemic.

In September 2009, as reports emerged from a Thai medical trial of an experimental HIV vaccine, newspaper headlines trumpeted a 'HIV breakthrough' (*Guardian* 24/09/2009). The trial, sponsored by the US Army and the US National Institute of Allergy and Infectious Diseases, involved 16,000 volunteers between the ages of 18 and 30 (NIAID 2009). There have been questions about the ethics of the trial; it involved healthy volunteers and the US agencies involved chose to run the trial in a 'Third World' country. However, the results were 'statistically significant', suggesting that the vaccine, a combination of two previously failed vaccines, offers a 31 percent lower chance of infection. The moderate protection it offers makes it a qualified success, because cutting sub-Saharan infections by a third would save literally hundreds of thousands of lives. At the same time, even if this vaccine were eventually to become available commercially, in a form modified to suit sub-Saharan

African purposes, the same problems associated with ARV rollout would quickly become apparent: sub-Saharan Africa's current lack of health-care infrastructure and medical personnel has the potential to undermine the efficacy of any new vaccine.

Male circumcision, while less headline-grabbing than a vaccine, has also been found to offer some protection against HIV. A US Centre for Disease Control (CDC 2008) literature survey has found that the procedure offers 'substantial protective effect' and can reduce the relative risk of HIV infection by 44 percent. A UNAIDS (2008c) report puts this figure higher, claiming circumcision can reduce the risk of infection by up to 60 percent. Studies have also shown that circumcision protects against a number of additional sexually-transmitted infections (CDC 2008). Countries in Africa and Asia demonstrating high levels of male circumcision show lower rates of HIV-prevalence than countries in which circumcision rates are low.[1] Consequently, the WHO and UNAIDS have suggested a scaling-up of circumcision in parts of Africa where it is currently less common (UNAIDS 2008c). However, there are gender and health-care considerations: there is little evidence to suggest that circumcision offers any protection to the sexual partners of circumcized men (CDC 2008), and problems with healthcare infrastructure could potentially restrict effective rollout. Circumcisions undertaken by traditional practitioners in South Africa's Eastern Cape Province have resulted in gangrene, amputations and even deaths. Between 1995 and 2008, more than 300 teenage boys have died as a result of botched circumcisions in the province and a further 6,000 have been hospitalized (Vincent 2008).

Without the prospect of a 'magic bullet', effective governance offers the only real bulwark against HIV/AIDS. In this respect, general health-care infrastructure is crucial. The fact that trained medical professionals are in such short supply largely negates the possibility of comprehensive treatment. That 36 African countries have a shortage of trained doctors, nurses and midwives is indicative of an overall crisis in health-care (WHO 2006a). The most telling statistic of all is that Africa, confronted with 24 percent of the global burden of disease, employs just 3 percent of the world's healthcare workers (WHO 2006a). This factor on its own can plausibly account for the continent's inability to check HIV/AIDS. Even if ARVs were provided free of charge, coverage would remain low due to poor distribution networks. Poverty is clearly an issue in this respect and it is therefore imperative that international donors focus more funding on the creation and maintenance of healthcare infrastructure. Furthermore, developed countries like the United Kingdom, where 33 percent of resident doctors received their training abroad, should refrain from creating circumstances that encourage the 'poaching' of medical personnel from developing countries. At the same time, the fact that only Botswana and The Gambia have achieved the 2001 Abuja Declaration target of allocating 15 percent of total government expenditure to health also means that African political elites have yet to prioritize healthcare spending (African Union 2007). Critics decrying the *cause célèbre* status of HIV/AIDS are correct in at least one aspect – more funds should be allocated to healthcare systems generally.

Tied closely to deficiencies in the overall healthcare infrastructure of sub-Saharan Africa is the role played by traditional healers in 'taking up the slack'. While the ratio of medical doctor to patient is often as high as 1:20,000, the ratio of traditional healer to patient is often as low as 1:200 (WHO 2002). Add to this the fact that approximately 80 percent of people living in sub-Saharan Africa employ the services of traditional healers (WHO 2002, 2008b), and there is a clear logic for formalizing the role of such practitioners in the provision of healthcare. However, this is problematic for a number of reasons. The lack of qualified medical personnel is a problem that must be addressed; it cannot be covered up by formally incorporating traditional practitioners into the healthcare system. Furthermore, the 'witchcraft paradigm' of disease, evident across much of sub-Saharan Africa (Evans-Pritchard 1937; Ngubane 1977; Beidelman 1963; Beattie 1963; Buxton 1963; Ashforth 2001, 2002, 2005; Ingstad 1990; Niehaus 2001; Meyer-Weitz *et al* 1998; Thomas 2008; Liddell *et al* 2005), is significantly at odds with many aspects of prevention and treatment programmes. In this cosmology, many diseases are understood in terms of malevolent forces acting against victims. Illnesses can only be abrogated, so the belief goes, if these forces are contained and combated by traditional healers. The qualifications necessary to become a traditional healer are somewhat arcane and difficult to quantify but nevertheless require a measure of 'calling' to the profession, usually entailing visions or dreams. Traditional remedies are, likewise, frequently 'revealed' to practitioners in dreams. Under such circumstances, the only way for traditional healers to be truly effective in HIV/AIDS management is for the sector to be encouraged to press patients to be tested by biomedical practitioners; a truly reciprocal exchange of ideas is difficult to envisage. Many African traditional medicines prescribed for the treatment of HIV/AIDS have been shown to be, at best, non-toxic. Estimates from South Africa alone suggest that thousands of people die every year as a result of the consumption of toxic traditional remedies (Popat *et al* 2001). Furthermore, the 'witchcraft paradigm' of illness makes the notion of sexually-transmitted diseases difficult to square because witchcraft is usually viewed as victim-specific. Such interpretations undermine 'safer sex' messages.

Until the 'magic bullet' is found, identifying effective prevention strategies will remain crucial to stemming the tide of HIV/AIDS. The role of condoms and notions of 'safer sex' are central in this regard. Pronouncements by high-ranking members of the Catholic Church, including the Pope, together with utterances from religiously-motivated political figures such as former US President George W. Bush, Ugandan President Yoweri Museveni and Ugandan First Lady Janet Museveni, that condoms are ineffective in preventing the spread of HIV/AIDS, that they promote increased levels of promiscuity and that their use puts people's lives at risk, has generated a significant degree of controversy. According to this perspective, a 'social vaccine' based on the promulgation of the largely Christian moral values of abstinence and fidelity is most likely to produce reductions in HIV prevalence. However, the supporting evidence for the efficacy of abstinence education is highly contested. While the newly-pioneered Thai vaccine outlined above diminishes the risk of infection by 31 percent, and circumcision might cut the risk to men by as much as 60 percent, condoms, when used properly are up to 90 percent effective in preventing the spread of HIV (Hearst and Chen 2004). Thailand's '100 percent programme', which mandated the use of condoms in brothels, is a demonstration of how effective governance can be in reducing risk. On such evidence, the promotion of increased condom use thus has to be at the heart of any HIV/AIDS education campaign. Given the importance of American funding in shaping the direction of treatment and prevention initiatives in sub-Saharan Africa via the auspices of PEPFAR, secular HIV/AIDS activists were reassured when President Barack Obama declared that 'best practice, not ideology' would henceforth determine US strategy on HIV/AIDS (Walker 2009).

While improved healthcare infrastructure lies at the centre of attempts to treat HIV/AIDS sufferers, the ready availability of proven-quality pharmaceuticals are a further prerequisite. The price of AIDS-related drugs is clearly an important element in determining ARV coverage. As generic drugs have flooded the market, so prices for first-line therapies have tumbled, from approximately $10,000 per year in the mid-1990s to just over $100 in 2007. However, the major pharmaceutical companies have fought a determined rearguard action in the interests of clawing back their control over medical patents. The Trade Related Aspects of Intellectual Property Rights (TRIPS) agreement, which forms part of the WTO framework, offers significant levels of protection to drugs patented after

1995. While 'flexibilities' in the TRIPS regime allow countries to issue compulsory licences in the case of public health emergencies, lobbying from so-called 'Big Pharma' has ensured heavy diplomatic pressure from the US being exerted on 'recalcitrant' countries like Brazil that have attempted to utilize these flexibilities. While the pharmaceutical industry has largely lost control over first-line therapies, companies manufacturing generics will find it increasingly difficult to copy and manufacture the newer, less toxic 'second-line' therapies developed after 1995. If this is the case, then access to these drugs, which becomes necessary once patients build up resistance to first-line therapies, will be severely restricted in regions like sub-Saharan Africa. The governance of the international trading regime is crucial where determining access to drugs is concerned and it is important that the safeguards protecting the interests of developing countries are robust. The stalling of the Doha Round has allowed the US in particular to increasingly circumvent TRIPS and to push instead for TRIPS-plus conditionality when negotiating free trade agreements with developing countries. While the WTO has its critics, the safeguards inherent in TRIPS, if countries felt free to apply them, would go a long way towards ensuring universal provision of ARVs.

More must be done to address the gender-based aspects of HIV/AIDS. Kofi Annan (2002) was correct in describing the African AIDS crisis as having a 'woman's face'. The fact that women suffer disproportionately from HIV/AIDS in sub-Saharan Africa is without doubt; of those infected with HIV, 60 percent are women. However, even these statistics do not represent adequately the full extent of the disparity between the risk posed by HIV to men and women. Adolescent girls and young women are especially vulnerable due to high levels of intergenerational sex and sexual violence. In South Africa, amongst 15 to 24 year olds, almost 90 percent of new infections occur in women (UNAIDS 2008a), while in the 20 to 29 year old demographic, HIV incidence is more than six times higher amongst women than men in the same cohort (UNAIDS 2008a). High levels of sexual violence across the continent also serve to undermine prevention efforts such as 'safer sex' messages and abstinence programmes – if women cannot control sexual access to their bodies, then such prevention efforts are largely meaningless. Thousands of women and young girls in conflict zones like the Democratic Republic of Congo and Sudan have been subjected to physical and sexual assaults, putting them at increased risk of contracting HIV. Yet such violence is prevalent outside of conflict zones too, with as many as 500,000 rapes being perpetuated in South Africa every year (SAPS 2005). Child victims account for nearly 40 percent of this total. While it is true that women are physiologically more susceptible to HIV/AIDS, such rape statistics belie a complex quandary for those charged with containing HIV/AIDS. South Africa, with its liberal constitution and Equality Courts is proof that formal statements and legal niceties can often have little impact in affecting gender equality 'on the ground'. A far greater engagement with the realities of entrenched gender hierarchies must be adopted as a prerequisite for any HIV/AIDS prevention programme. Once again, political leadership is important and, in this instance, noticeably lacking. The 'traditional values' reemphasized by leaders like President Museveni and current South African President Jacob Zuma arguably serve to entrench gender hierarchies. Museveni's encouragement of early marriages for women and Zuma's polygamy and advocation of rites like 'virginity testing' all serve to reinforce the hierarchical nature of existing gender relations. Until gender equality is recognized as an end in itself, as outlined in the Millennium Development Goals (Goal 3), it is likely that the pandemic will continue unabated.

In the fight against HIV/AIDS, African political leadership is crucial. President Museveni represents Africa's most celebrated champion in the fight against HIV/AIDS and he has cemented his position as a global statesman in this respect, travelling to the US in November 2007 and holding meetings with George W Bush, the then Secretary of State, Condeleezza Rice, and the Speaker of the House, Nancy Pelosi. While his motives have been brought into question (Tumushabe 2006) and the full extent of the 'Ugandan miracle' has been queried (Allen, T. 2005), Museveni has undoubtedly been successful in forcing Ugandans to engage with many of the realities of HIV/AIDS. In this respect, as an African statesman, he is something of a rarity. Political leadership in the area of HIV/AIDS, especially in the early stages of the pandemic, has varied between cynical attempts to increase aid, as was the case in Malawi and Cameroon during the 1980s, to apathy, as manifest in countries like Nigeria, and outright AIDS-scepticism, as evident in South Africa. In this respect, the political leadership of former South African President Thabo Mbeki has been well documented. The failure of Mbeki's government to throw its weight behind attempts to combat HIV/AIDS has resulted in needless suffering. It is apparent that, in many respects, Africa is in need of more home-grown champions against HIV/AIDS.

In the absence of a cure or an effective vaccine, the work to contain and eventually roll back HIV/AIDS in sub-Saharan Africa must continue. In this sense, managing HIV/AIDS is simply part of the broader development framework expressed by the Millennium Development Goals (combating HIV/AIDS forms part of Goal 6). Poverty and communicable diseases go hand-in-hand, as is evidenced by the fact that in Africa, 72 percent of deaths are caused by communicable disease and complications arising from pregnancy and childbirth (WHO 2006b). In Europe and the US, the majority of deaths are caused by non-communicable illnesses such as cancer and heart disease. In this respect at least, Thabo Mbeki has been largely correct. HIV/AIDS is a disease of poverty. It is also a problem for political economists. The key international donors PEPFAR, Global Fund and MAP cannot be seen as the solution to the HIV/AIDS crisis; they are, in many respects, only treating the symptoms. Robust political leadership, especially on the part of African political elites, is imperative. Leaders can show the way by following the path set by Botswana and The Gambia in devoting 15 percent of government spending to healthcare. Political leaders can also work to ensure that gender equality becomes the norm both in statute and in practice, thereby addressing the gender hierarchies largely responsible for the spread of HIV/AIDS. Fundamentally, combating HIV/AIDS is about ensuring that, rather than it being pigeon-holed simply as a health issue and a 'natural disaster', it is understood for what it really is: a breakdown of governance from which lessons must be learned.

Notes

Introduction

1 Somewhat confusingly, the Meredith text is published under different titles in the United States and the United Kingdom. The US version is published as *The Fate of Africa: From the Hopes of Freedom to the Heart of Despair – A History of Fifty Years of Independence* (Meredith 2006b).
2 Yaws is a disease of the skin, bone and cartilage affecting people living in tropical areas. Whilst not fatal, it can lead to disability and disfigurement. Extensive measures were made to control it during the 1950s and 1960s, when programmes were rolled out in 46 countries by the WHO and UNICEF (WHO 2009a).
3 This was prior to the complex socio-political and economic meltdown that overtook Zimbabwe post-2000.
4 Traditional remedies are frequently extremely costly. In 2006, the controversial herbal 'cure' for HIV/AIDS, *uBhejane* (see Chapter 5) retailed at R170 ($22) for a three-day course, equating to an outlay of R2000 ($262) per month. ARVs were, and continue to be, free of charge (*Financial Mail* 05/05/2006). To put the cost of *uBhejane* into perspective, in 2004, even after the introduction of a minimum wage, the average South African domestic worker struggled to 'take home' more than R1000 ($131) per month (Hertz 2004). Similarly, on the onset of visible symptoms of HIV/AIDS in an individual, the resultant urgent interventions to placate displeased ancestors can also be extremely expensive, with ancestral feasts and extensive consultations with traditional healers consuming a significant proportion of a family's income (Ashforth 2001).

Chapter 1   Sex and Disease: A Historical Perspective

1 Gonorrhoea, conversely, was well known across much of the ancient world; Leviticus provides a case-closed description (Leviticus Chapter 15, King James Version; see also Bollet 2004), and the disease, so named by Galen, was also described by Hippocrates, Plato and Aristotle (Barlow 2006).
2 Other diseases from the 'New World' are thought to include yaws, hepatitis, encephalitis, polio and certain strains of tuberculosis (Crosby 2004).

Chapter 2   The Origins of HIV/AIDS

1 Gabon, Equatorial Guinea, Cameroon, and the Democratic Republic of Congo.
2 HIV-1 is the more virulent of the strains and is responsible for the global HIV/AIDS pandemic. HIV-2 is far less infectious in its early stages and is slower in destroy the victim's immune system. HIV-2 remains largely confined to West Africa.

3 As a retrovirus, HIV belongs to the same 'family' of viruses that cause leukaemia in humans and other mammals. Retroviruses are also categorized as 'lentiviruses', because they are slow acting (WHO 2000).
4 A normal CD4 count is between 800–1500.

Chapter 3   Gender, Violence and the Spread of HIV/AIDS

1 Post-exposure prophylaxis (PEP) is a short-term ARV treatment designed to reduce the likelihood of HIV infection after possible exposure ie unprotected, sexual intercourse, rape, or occupational hazards such as needlesticks (WHO 2010a).
2 Zuma was found not guilty in May 2006, the court ruling that the sexual contact between the defendant and the alleged victim was consensual.
3 Necklacing is a form of lynching carried out by perpetrators forcing a tire filled with petrol over the victim's shoulders and then setting it alight.

Chapter 4   Policymaking, Dissidents and Denialists

1 Readers interested in this debate are encouraged to read A. F. Chalmers' (1999) *What Is This Thing Called Science?*
2 http://www.duesberg.com/about/bribepd.html

Chapter 6   The International Response: Multilateral and Unilateral Approaches

1 The WHO Prequalification of Medicines Project was established in 2001 with the aim of improving access to drugs designed to treat HIV/AIDS, malaria, and tuberculosis. The prequalification process 'aims to ensure that diagnostics, medicines and vaccines for high-burden diseases meet global standards of quality, safety and efficacy, in order to optimize use of health resources and improve health outcomes' (WHO 2010b).
2 In January 2010, the Bill and Melinda Gates Foundation (2010) announced funding of $10 billion to be spread over ten years.

Chapter 7   Morality, Behavioural Change and the Search for a 'Social Vaccine'

1 The President's Emergency Plan for AIDS Relief (PEPFAR) was introduced in 2003 by then President George W Bush. Initially allocated a budget of $15 billion to be spread over five years, the initiative was renewed in 2008, with a budget of $48 billion (Chapter 6).
2 Catholic Relief Services, together with the Catholic Medical Mission Board (CMMB), the Institute of Human Virology (IHV) at the University of Maryland, USA, Constella Futures, and Interchurch Medical Assistance (IMA), established AIDSRelief in 2003. The programme is operational in nine countries: Guyana, Haiti, Kenya, Nigeria, Rwanda, South Africa, Tanzania, Uganda

and Zambia, and was allocated a budget of $371 million, courtesy of PEPFAR, in 2004 (CRS 2008b).

3 Museveni came to power in 1986 after a lengthy military campaign against the sitting President, Milton Obote. Initially viewed as a 'renaissance' African leader in the West, his reputation has been somewhat tarnished by his determination to cling to power. He courted controversy by standing in the 2006 presidential election after promising in his 2001 campaign to step down once that term ended. He has been repeatedly accused of electoral fraud and the persecution of political opponents. His current term expires in 2011 (ICTJ 2008).

4 By 2004 the Ugandan government estimated prevalence amongst 15–49 year olds to be 6.1 percent. By 2007, this figure had risen to 6.7 percent (Ugandan Government 2008).

Chapter 8   Governance, the International Trading System and Access to Antiretrovirals

1 The General Agreement on Tariffs and Trade (GATT), established to regulate international trade and cut tariff barriers, was born out of the Bretton Woods Negotiations held just before the end of the Second World War. It was in effect from 1947 until 1995 when it was replaced by the WTO.

2 Compulsory licensing: when a government allows for the production of a patented product or process without the consent of the patent holder.

3 As of February 2010, the bilateral Free Trade Agreement negotiations between the US and Thailand remain 'dormant' (Cooper 2010).

4 International dollars (I$) are derived by dividing local currency units by an estimate of their purchasing power parity compared to the US dollar (WHO 2008c).

Conclusion

1 The age at which circumcision takes place is important. A 2007 study undertaken amongst Xhosa initiates in South Africa's Eastern Cape Province showed that only 12 percent of respondents were circumcized prior to sexual debut. In the year preceding circumcision, nearly 20 percent had been diagnosed with a sexually-transmitted disease (Peltzer *et al* 2008).

Bibliography

ActionAid (2009) 'Hate Crimes: The Rise of "Corrective" Rape in South Africa', Report, March <http://www.actionaid.org.uk/doc_lib/correctiveraperep_final. pdf>.

Adetunji, J. and Bos, E. R. (2006) 'Levels and Trends in Mortality in Sub-Saharan Africa: An Overview', in Jamison, D. T., Feachem, R. G., Makgoba, M. W., Bos, E. R., Baingana, F. K., Hofman, K. J. and Rogo, K. O. (eds) *Disease and Mortality in Sub-Saharan Africa*, Second Edition (Washington DC: World Bank).

Adinkrah, M. (2004) 'Witchcraft Accusations and Female Homicide Victimization in Contemporary Ghana', *Violence Against Women*, 10(4): 325–56.

African Union (2007) 'African Health Strategy: 2007–2015', 3rd Ordinary Session of the Conference of African Union of Ministers of Health (CAMH3), 9–13 April, Sandton Convention Centre, Johannesburg, South Africa.

AIDSTruth (2008) 'AIDS Denialists Lie about More than HIV: Deception and Duplicity among the "Dissidents"', AIDSTruth Report, August <http://www.aid-struth.org/new/sites/default/files/lying-denialists_0.pdf>.

Alcorn, K. (2007) 'Brazil Issues Compulsory License on Efavirenz', AIDSMap News, 7 May <http://www.aidsmap.com/en/news/0550CE62-3F90-4603-932C-EF69E1B4485D.asp>.

Allen, J. (2005) 'Accepting the Whitsitt Society Award', *The Whitsitt Journal*, 13(2), Fall.

Allen, P. L. (2000) *The Wages of Sin* (Chicago and London: University of Chicago Press).

Allen, T. (2005) 'AIDS and Evidence: Interrogating Some Ugandan Myths', *Journal of Biosocial Science*, 38(1): 7–28.

Alliance India (2006) 'Indian Government has No Plans for Second-Line Anti-retrovirals', International HIV/AIDS Alliance, December <http://www.aidsal-liance.org/sw43893.asp>.

Altman, D. (1988) 'The Impact of AIDS in the Developed World', *British Medical Bulletin*, 44(1): 170–82.

Amnesty International (2005) 'Rape as a Tool of War', Fact Sheet, 25 August.

Andrews, P. (2007) 'Democracy Stops at My Front Door: Obstacles to Gender Equality in South Africa', *Loyola University Chicago International Law Review*, 5(1): 15–28.

Andrews, P. (2009) 'Who's Afraid of Polygamy? Exploring the Boundaries of Family, Equality and Custom in South Africa', *University of Utah Law Review*, No. 2, 351.

Anglican Church (2008) 'The Anglican Communion', Information Pamphlet, February.

Annan, K. (2002) 'In Africa, AIDS has a Woman's Face', *New York Times*, 29 December.

Anonymous (2002) 'Castro Hlongwane, Caravans, Cats, Geese, Foot and Mouth and Statistics: HIV/AIDS and the Struggle for the Humanisation of the African', Pamphlet.

ASA (2008) 'Ubhejane Product/TAC/10649', Ruling of the Advertising Standards Authority of South Africa, 8 April.

Ashforth, A. (2001) 'AIDS, Witchcraft, and the Problem of Power in Post-Apartheid South Africa', Institute for Advanced Studies, School of Social Sciences, Occasional Paper, Number 10, May.

Ashforth, A. (2002) 'An Epidemic of Witchcraft? The Implications of AIDS for the Post-Apartheid State', *African Studies*, 61(1): 121–43.

Ashforth, A. (2005) *Witchcraft, Violence, and Democracy in South Africa* (Chicago: University of Chicago Press).

Baker, B. J., Armelagos, G. J., Becker, M. J., Brothwell, D., Drusini, A., Geise, M. C., Kelley, M. A., Moritoto, I., Morris, A. G., Nurse, G. T., Powell, M. L., Rothschild, B. M. and Saunders, S. R. (1988) 'The Origin and Antiquity of Syphilis: Paleopathological Diagnosis and Interpretation', *Current Anthropology*, 29(5): 703–37.

Balasubramaniam, K. (2002) 'Access to Medicines: Patents, Prices and Public Policy – Consumer Perspectives', in Drahos, P. and Mayne, R. (eds) *Global Intellectual Property Rights: Knowledge, Access and Development* (Basingstoke: Palgrave Macmillan).

Barker, J. (2006) *Agincourt: The King, the Campaign, the Battle* (London: Abacus).

Barlow, D. (2006) *Sexually Transmitted Infections: The Facts* (Oxford: Oxford University Press).

Barnett, T. and Whiteside, A. (2006) *AIDS in the Twenty-First Century: Disease and Globalization* (Basingstoke: Palgrave Macmillan).

Bass, E. (2005) 'Fighting to Close the Condom Gap in Uganda', *The Lancet*, 365, 26 March–1 April: 1127–8.

Batsell, J. (2005) 'AIDS, Politics and NGOs in Zimbabwe', in Patterson, A. S. (ed.) *The African State and the AIDS Crisis* (London: Ashgate).

BBC (2004) 'SA Leader Urges Virginity Tests', BBC News, 23 September <http://news.bbc.co.uk/1/hi/world/africa/3683210.stm>.

Beattie, J. (1963) 'Sorcery in Bunyoro', in Middleton, J. and Winter, E. H. (eds) *Witchcraft and Sorcery in East Africa* (London: Routledge and Kegan Paul), pp. 27–56.

Beidelman, T. O. (1963) 'Witchcraft in Ukaguru', in Middleton, J. and Winter, E. H. (eds) *Witchcraft and Sorcery in East Africa* (London: Routledge and Kegan Paul), pp. 57–98.

Beinart, W. and Hughes, L. (2007) *Environment and Empire* (Oxford: Oxford University Press).

Bendavid, E. and Bhattacharya, J. (2009) 'The President's Emergency Plan for AIDS Relief in Africa: An Evaluation of Outcomes', *Annals of Internal Medicine*, 150(10): 688–95.

Bhana, K., Gerntholtz, L., Hurt, K., Meeson, A. and Vetten, L. (2004) 'Health and Hope in Our Hands Addressing HIV and AIDS in the Aftermath of Rape and Woman Abuse', AIDS Law Project Guide.

Bialy, H. (2004) *Oncogenes, Aneuploidy and AIDS: A Scientific Life and Times of Peter H Duesberg* (Berkeley: North Atlantic Books).

Bill and Melinda Gates Foundation (2001) 'Bill & Melinda Gates Foundation Pledges $100 Million Toward $550 Million AIDS Vaccine Goal', Press Release, 27 January <http://www.gatesfoundation.org/press-releases/Pages/international-aids-vaccine-initiative-010127.aspx>.

Bill and Melinda Gates Foundation (2010) 'Bill and Melinda Gates Pledge $10 Billion in Call for Decade of Vaccines', Press Release, 29 January <http://www.gates-

foundation.org/press-releases/Pages/decade-of-vaccines-wec-announcement-100129.aspx>.

Blaikie, W. G. (2009) *The Personal Life of David Livingstone Chiefly From His Unpublished Journals and Correspondence in the Possession of His Family* (Salt Lake City: Project Gutenberg).

Boesten, J. and Poku, N. K. (eds) (2009) *Gender and HIV/AIDS: Critical Perspectives from the Developing World* (Farnham: Ashgate).

Boler, T. and Ingham, R. (2007) 'The Abstinence Debate: Condoms, the President's Emergency Plan for AIDS Relief (PEPFAR) and Ideology', *Action Aid Policy and Research*: Issue 4.

Bollet, A. J. (2004) *Plagues and Poxes: The Impact of Human History on Epidemic Disease* (New York: Demos).

Brant, J. (2003) 'Robbing the Poor to Pay the Rich?', Oxfam Briefing Paper, Number 56, November.

Brink, A. (2000) *Debating AZT: Mbeki and the AIDS Drugs Controversy* (Pietermaritzburg: Open Books).

Burr, T., Hyman, J. M. and Myers, G. (2001) 'The Origin of Acquired Immune Deficiency Syndrome: Darwinian or Lamarckian', *The Royal Society, Philosophical Transactions B*, 356(1410): 877–87.

Bush, G. W. (2004) 'State of the Union Address', Washington DC <http://georgewbushwhitehouse.archives.gov/news/releases/2004/01/20040120-7.html>.

Buxton, J. (1963) 'Mandari Witchcraft', in Middleton, J. and Winter, E. H. (eds) *Witchcraft and Sorcery in East Africa* (London: Routledge and Kegan Paul).

Cabral, A. J. R. (1993) 'AIDS in Africa: Can the Hospitals Cope?', *Health Policy and Planning*, 8(2): 157–60.

Cahn, N. R. (2006) 'Poor Children: Child Witches and Child Soldiers in Sub-Saharan Africa', GWU Law School Public Law Research Paper, Number 177.

Caldwell, J. C., Caldwell, P. and Quiggin, P. (1989) 'The Social Context of AIDS in Sub-Saharan Africa', *Population and Development Review*, 15(2): 185–234.

Caraël, M. (2006) 'Twenty Years of Intervention and Controversy', in Denis, P. and Becker, C. (eds) *The HIV/AIDS Epidemic in Sub-Saharan Africa in a Historical Perspective* (Paris: Academia-Bruylant), pp. 29–40.

Caraël, M. and Glynn, J. R. (2007) 'HIV Infection in Young Adults in Africa: Context, Risks and Opportunities for Prevention', in Caraël, M. and Glynn, J. R. (eds) *HIV, Resurgent Infections and Population Change in Africa* (Dordrecht: Springer).

Carey, J. (2006) 'Exxon's Climate Denial – Again', *Business Week*, 22 May <http://www.businessweek.com/investing/green_business/archives/2007/05/exxons_climate.html>.

Caritas (2008) 'Caritas AIDS Response Around the World', HIV/AIDS Response <http://www.caritas.org/activities/hiv_aids/sinethemba_a_caritas_response_to_aids.html?cnt=464>.

Carstens, P. A. (2003) 'The Cultural Defence in Criminal Law: South African Perspectives', 17th International Conference of the International Society for the Reform of Criminal Law, The Hague, August 24–28.

CDC (2008) 'Male Circumcision and Risk for HIV Transmission and Other Health Conditions: Implications for the United States', Centre for Disease Control and Prevention, CDC HIV/AIDS Science Facts.

CDC (2009) 'Leading Causes of Death', Centre for Disease Control and Prevention Fact Sheet <http://www.cdc.gov/nchs/FASTATS/lcod.htm>.

CEFIKS (2009) 'Mission Statement', Centre for Indigenous Knowledge Systems (CEFIKS) <http://www.cfiks.org/>.

Chamberlain, M. E. (1999) *The Scramble for Africa* (London: Longman).

Chalmers, A. F. (1999) *What Is This Thing Called Science?* (Milton Keynes: Open University Press).

Charlesworth, H. (1995) 'Human Rights as Men's Rights', in Peters, J. and Wolper, A. (eds) *Women's Rights Human Rights* (London: Routledge), pp. 103–13.

Chattoe-Brown, A. and Bitunda, A. (2006) 'Reproductive Health Commodity Security: Uganda Country Case Study', Department for International Development (UK) and the Netherlands Ministry of Foreign Affairs.

Chien, C. V. (2007) 'HIV/AIDS Drugs for Sub-Saharan Africa: How Do Brand and Generic Supply Compare?', Santa Clara University School of Law, Legal Studies Research Papers Series Working Paper, Number 07-41, August.

Chigwedere, P., Seage III, G. R., Gruskin, S. and Lee, T. (2008) 'Estimating the Lost Benefits of Antiretroviral Drug Use in South Africa', *Journal of Acquired Immune Deficiency Syndrome*, 49(4): 410–15.

Chirac, P. and Torreele, E. (2006) 'Global Framework on Essential Health R&D', *The Lancet*, 367, 13 May: 1560–1.

Chopra, M., Kendall, C., Hill, Z., Schaay, N., Nkonki, L. L. and Doherty, T. M. (2006) '"Nothing New": Responses to the Introduction of Antiretroviral Drugs in South Africa', *AIDS*, 20(15): 1975–86.

Clinton Foundation (2009) 'President Clinton, Pfizer, and Mylan Announce New Agreements to Lower Prices of Medicines for Patients with Drug-Resistant HIV in Developing Countries', Press Release, 6 August <http://www.clinton-foundation.org/news/news-media/press-release-president-clinton-pfizer-and-mylan-announce-new-agreements-to-lower-prices-of-medicines-for-patients-with-drug-resistant-hiv-in-developing-countries>.

Clinton, W. J. (1991) 'A New Covenant for American Security', Speech, Georgetown University, Democratic Leadership Council, 12 December <http://www.ndol.org/ndol_ci.cfm?kaid=128&subid=174&contentid=25053>.

Clinton, W. J. (2001) 'The Diana, Princess of Wales Lecture on AIDS', London, National AIDS Trust, 13 December.

Cohen, S. A. (2003) 'Beyond Slogans: Lessons from Uganda's Experience with ABC and HIV/AIDS', *Reproductive Health Matters*, 12(23): 132–5.

Commission on Health Research for Development (1990) *Health Research: Essential Link to Equity in Development* (New York: Oxford University Press).

Conlan, M. F. (2008) 'Lobbying Spending Hits New Record', *America's Pharmacist*, June <http://www.ncpanet.org/pdf/notes/amrxjune08notes.pdf>.

Coomaraswamy, R. (1997) 'Report of the Special Rapporteur on Violence against Women, its Causes and Consequences', Report on the Mission of the Special Rapporteur to South Africa on the Issue of Rape in the Community, 11–18 October.

Cooper, F. and Stoler, A. L. (1989) 'Tensions of Empire: Colonial Control and Visions of Rule', *American Ethnologist*, 16(4): 609–21.

Cooper, W. H. (2010) 'Free Trade Agreements: Impact on US Trade and Implications for US Trade Policy', Congressional Research Service Report for Congress, 23 February.

Copson, R. W. (2003) 'AIDS in Africa: Issue Brief for Congress', Congressional Research Service, 24 April <http://fpc.state.gov/documents/organization/20243.pdf>.

Correa, C. (2007) 'Guidelines for the Examination of Pharmaceutical Patents: Developing a Public Health Perspective', ICTSD, UNCTAD and WHO Working Paper, January.

Cribb, J. (2001) 'The Origin of Acquired Immune Deficiency Syndrome: Can Science Afford to Ignore It?', *The Royal Society, Philosophical Transactions B*, 356(1410): 935–8.

Crosby, A. W. (2003) *America's Forgotten Pandemic*, New Edition (Cambridge: Cambridge University Press).

Crosby, A. W. (2004) *Ecological Imperialism: The Biological Expansion of Europe 900–1900*, Second Edition (Cambridge: Cambridge University Press).

Crowell, B. (1998) *Newtonian Physics* (California: Fullerton).

CRS (2008a) 'Promising Practises II: HIV and AIDS Integrated Programming', Catholic Relief Services, March.

CRS (2008b) 'Catholic Relief Services AIDSRelief Milestone', Catholic Relief Services Press Release, 23 July.

Cullinan, K. and Thom, A. (eds) (2009) *The Virus, Vitamins and Vegetables: The South African HIV/AIDS Mystery* (Sunnyside: Jacana).

Culshaw, R. V. (2007) *Science Sold Out: Does HIV Really Cause AIDS?* (Berkeley: North Atlantic Books).

Curtis, T. (1992) 'The Origin of AIDS', *Rolling Stone Magazine*, 19 March.

Davies, J. N. P. (1956) 'The History of Syphilis in Uganda', *World Health Organisation Bulletin*, 15(6): 1041–55.

De Cock, K. M. (2001) 'Epidemiology and the Emergence of Human Immuno-deficiency Virus and Acquired Immune Deficiency Syndrome', *The Royal Society, Philosophical Transactions B*, 356(1410): 795–8.

Delius, P. and Glaser, C. (2004) 'The Myths of Polygamy: A History of Extra-Marital and Multi-Partnership Sex in South Africa', *South African Historical Journal*, 50(1): 84–114.

Department of Health (2007) 'HIV/AIDS/STI Strategic Plan for South Africa 2007–2011' <http://www.doh.gov.za/docs/misc/stratplan-f.html>.

Department of Health (2009) '2008 National Antenatal Sentinel HIV & Syphilis Prevalence Survey', South African Government Report, September.

De Waal, A. (2006) *AIDS and Power: Why There is No Political Crisis – Yet.* (London/ New York: Zed).

Doctors for Life (2006) 'South Africa – AIDS "Cure", Ubhejane, Fails Test', Press Release, 13 November.

Doezema, J. (2001) 'Ouch! Western Feminists' "Wounded Attachment" to the "Third World Prostitute"', *Feminist Review*, 67, Spring: 16–38.

Drahos, P. (2002) 'Negotiating Intellectual Property Rights: Between Coercion and Dialogue', in Drahos, P. and Mayne, R. (eds) *Global Intellectual Property Rights: Knowledge, Access and Development* (Basingstoke: Palgrave Macmillan), pp. 161–82.

Drucker, E., Alcabes, P. G. and Marx, P. A. (2001) 'The Injection Century: Massive Unsterile Injections and the Emergence of Human Pathogens', *The Lancet*, 358: 1989–92.

Duesberg, P. H. (1987) 'Retroviruses as Carcinogens and Pathogens: Expectations and Reality', *Cancer Research*, 47(5): 1199–220.

Duesberg, P. H. (1988) 'HIV is Not the Cause of AIDS', *Science*, 241, 29 July: 514–17.

Duesberg, P. H. (1989) 'Defective Viruses and AIDS', Correspondence, *Nature*, 340, 17 August: 515.

Duesberg, P. H. (1991) 'Duesberg on AIDS and HIV', Correspondence, *Nature*, 350, 7 March: 10.

Duesberg, P. H. (1992) 'Questions about AIDS', Correspondence, *Nature*, 358, 2 July: 10.

Duesberg, P. H. (1996) *Inventing the AIDS Virus* (Washington DC: Regnery).

Dunkle, K. L., Jewkes, R. K., Brown, H. C., Gray, G. E., McIntryre, J. A. and Harlow, S. D. (2004) 'Gender-Based Violence, Relationship Power, and Risk of HIV Infection in Women Attending Antenatal Clinics in South Africa', *The Lancet*, 363(9419): 1415–21.

Dunkle, K. L., Jewkes, R. K., Ndunad, M., Levinc, J., Jamab, N., Khuzwayob, N., Kosse, M. P. and Duvvury, N. (2006) 'Perpetration of Partner Violence and HIV Risk Behaviour among Young Men in the Rural Eastern Cape, South Africa', *AIDS*, 20(16): 2107–14.

Dunn, J. P., Krige, J. E. J., Wood, R., Bornman, P. C. and Terblanche, J. (1991) 'Colonic Complications after Toxic Tribal Enemas', *British Journal of Surgery*, 78(5): 545–8.

Eboko, F. (2005) 'Patterns of Mobilization: Political Culture in the Fight against AIDS', in Patterson, A. (ed.) *The African State and the AIDS Crisis* (Aldershot: Ashgate), pp. 37–58.

Elbe, S. (2006) 'Should HIV/AIDS be Securitized? The Ethical Dilemmas of Linking HIV/AIDS and Security', *International Studies Quarterly*, 50(1): 119–44.

England, R. (2007) 'Are We Spending Too Much on HIV?', *British Medical Journal*, 334(7589): 344.

EPHA (2006) 'What are the Leading Causes of Death in the EU?', European Public Health Alliance Fact Sheet <http://www.epha.org/a/2352>.

Evans-Pritchard, E. E. (1937) *Witchcraft, Oracles and Magic among the Azande* (Oxford: Clarendon Press).

Farber, C. (1989) 'Sins of Omission: The AZT Scandal', *Spin*, November.

Farber, C. (1991) 'AIDS: Words from The Front', *Spin*, April.

Farber, C. (1993) 'AZT is Death', *Spin*, August.

Farber, C. (1996) 'AZT on Trial', *Spin*, July.

Farber, C. (1997) 'The End of the End', *Spin*, April.

Farber, C. (1998) 'AZT Roulette: The Impossible Choices Facing HIV-positive Women', *Mothering*, September/October.

Farber, C. (2000) 'Science Fiction', *Gear Magazine*, March.

Farber, C. (2006a) 'Out of Control: AIDS and the Corruption of Medical Science', *Harper's Magazine*, 1 March.

Farber, C. (2006b) *Serious Adverse Events: An Uncensored History of AIDS* (New York: Melville House).

FDA (Food and Drug Administration) (2006) 'FDA Approves the First Once-a-Day Three-Drug Combination Tablet for Treatment of HIV-1', US Food and Drug Administration Press Release, July 12.

Federici, S. (2008) 'Witch-Hunting, Globalization, and Feminist Solidarity in Africa Today', *Journal of International Women's Studies*, 10(1): 21–35.

Financial Mail 05/05/2006.

Finer, L. B. (2007) 'Trends in Premarital Sex in the United States, 1954–2003', *Public Health Reports*, 122(1): 73–8.

Fink, C. and Reichenmiller, P. (2006) 'Tightening TRIPS: Intellectual Property Provisions of U.S. Free Trade Agreements', in Newfarmer, R. (ed.) *Trade, Doha and Development: A Window into the Issues* (Washington DC: The International Bank for Reconstruction and Development/The World Bank), pp. 289–303.

Fitzpatrick, J. (1994) 'The Use of International Human Rights Norms to Combat Violence against Women', in Cook, R. J. (ed.) *Human Rights of Women: National and International Perspectives* (Philadelphia: University of Pennsylvania Press), pp. 532–72.

Flint, A. G. (2009a) Group Interview, Healthcare Providers, Sophumelela Centre, East London (South Africa), 12 January.

Flint, A. G. (2009b) Interview, Director, Women in Partnership against AIDS, East London (South Africa), 13 January.

Flint, A. G. (2009c) Interview, Director, Ikhwezi Lokusa Wellness Centre, East London (South Africa), 14 January.

Flint, A. G. (2009d) Interview, HIV/AIDS Coordinator, Grahamstown Diocese, Church of the Province of South Africa, Queenstown (South Africa), 15 January.

Flint, A. G. (2009e) Interview, Director, Raphael Centre, Grahamstown (South Africa), 16 January.

Flint, A. G. (2009f) Interview, Focus Group, Teenage Youth Group, East London (South Africa), 17 January.

Flint, A. G. (2009g) Interview, Focus Group, Teenage Youth Group 2, East London (South Africa), 17 January.

Flint, A. G. (2009h) Interview, Focus Group, Teenage Youth Group 3, East London (South Africa), 17 January.

Flint, A. G. (2009i) Group Interview, Women Living with HIV/AIDS, East London (South Africa), 18 January.

Flint, A. G. (2009j) Photographs, East London, Grahamstown, Queenstown (South Africa), January.

Fourie, P. (2006) *The Political Management of HIV and AIDS in South Africa: One Burden too Many?* (Basingstoke: Palgrave Macmillan).

Fox, R. L. (2006) *The Classical World: An Epic History of Greece and Rome* (London: Penguin).

Frank, R. G. (1999) 'Effects of the Black Death in England: An Essay Review', *Journal of the History of Medicine*, 54: 596–605.

Fratkin, E. (1996) 'Traditional Medicine and Concepts of Healing among Samburu Pastoralists of Kenya', *Journal of Ethnobiology*, 16(1): 63–97.

Freund, B. (1998) *The Making of Contemporary Africa: The Development of African Society Since 1800* (Basingstoke: Palgrave Macmillan).

Fried, S. T. (2003) 'Violence against Women', *Health and Human Rights*, 6(2): 88–111.

Fiedrich, M. and Jellema, A. (2003) 'Literacy, Gender, and Social Agency: Adventures in Empowerment', Report for ActionAid UK, Department for International Development, September.

Gallo, R., Geffen, N., Gonsalves, G., Jeffreys, R., Kuritzkes, D. R., Mirken, B., Moore, J. P. and Safrit, J. T. (2006) 'Errors in Celia Farber's March 2006 Article in *Harper's Magazine*', Treatment Action Campaign.

GAO (Government Accountability Office) (2004) 'Global Health', US AIDS Coordinator Addressing Some Key Challenges to Expanding Treatment but Others Remain, GAO Report Number GAO-04-784, 12 July.

GAO (2006) 'New Drug Development – Science, Business, Regulatory, and Intellectual Property Issues Cited as Hampering Drug Development Efforts', Report by the United States Government Accountability Office, November.

Geffen, N. (2005) 'Echoes of Lysenko: State-Sponsored Pseudo-Science in South Africa', *Social Dynamics*, 31(2): 183–210.

Geffen, N. (2007) 'Encouraging Deadly Choices: AIDS Pseudo-Science in the Media', Centre for Social Science Research, Working Paper Number 182.

Gelfand, M. (1953) *Tropical Victory: An Account of the Influence of Medicine on the History of Southern Rhodesia* (Cape Town: Juta Press).

Gilbert, L. and Walker, L. (2002) 'HIV/AIDS in South Africa: An Overview', *Cad Saude Publica*, 18(3): 651–60.

Gilman, S. L. (1987) 'AIDS and Syphilis: The Iconography of Disease', *AIDS: Cultural Analysis/Cultural Activism*, 43, Winter: 87–107.

GlaxoSmithKline (2009a) 'Alnylam Joins GSK in Donating Intellectual Property to Patent Pool for Neglected Tropical Diseases', Press Release, 8 July <http://www.gsk.com/media/pressreleases/2009/2009_pressrelease_10071.htm>.

GlaxoSmithKline (2009b) 'GSK Announces New Commitments to Fight HIV/AIDS in Sub-Saharan Africa: Special Focus on Care and Treatment of Children', Press Release, 14 July <http://www.gsk.com/media/pressreleases/2009/2009_press-release_10073.htm>.

Gleick, P. (1992) 'Water and Conflict', Project on Environmental Change and Acute Conflict, Trudeau Centre for Peace and Conflict Studies, University of Toronto, Occasional Paper Series, Number 1, September.

Global Forum for Health Research (2006) 'Monitoring Financial Flows for Health Research 2005: Behind the Global Numbers', February.

Global Fund (2005) 'Questions on the Suspension of Grants in Uganda', Global Fund to Fight AIDS, Tuberculosis and Malaria, Press Release, 23 August <http://www.theglobalfund.org/content/pressreleases/pr_050824_faq.pdf>.

Global Fund (2007) 'The Global Fund: Who We Are, What We Do', Global Fund to Fight AIDS, Tuberculosis and Malaria, Brochure <http://www.theglobal-fund.org/documents/publications/brochures/whoweare/gf_brochure_07_full_high_en.pdf>.

Global Fund (2008) 'Reserve Bank of Zimbabwe Releases Global Fund Money', Global Fund to Fight AIDS, Tuberculosis and Malaria, Press Release, 7 November <http://www.theglobalfund.org/en/pressreleases/?pr=pr_081107>.

Global Fund (2010) 'About the Global Fund', Global Fund to Fight AIDS, Tuberculosis and Malaria <http://www.theglobalfund.org/en/about/>.

Global Health Council (2005) 'Faith in Action: Examining the Role of Faith Based Organisations in Addressing HIV/AIDS', Global Health Council <http://www.globalhealth.org/images/pdf/faith_in_action/faith_in_action_final.pdf>.

Glynn, J. R., Pönninghaus, J., Crampin, A. C., Sibande, F., Sichali, L., Nkhosa, P., Broadbent, P. and Fine, P. E. M. (2001) 'The Development of the HIV Epidemic in Karonga District, Malawi', *AIDS*, 15(15): 2025–9.

Golooba-Mutebi, F. and Tollman, S. M. (2007) 'Confronting HIV/AIDS in a South African Village: The Impact of Health-Seeking Behaviour', *Scandinavian Journal of Public Health*, 35(3): 175–80.

Goodstein, D. (2000) 'How Science Works', in *US Federal Judiciary Reference Manual on Evidence*, Second Edition (Washington DC: Federal Judicial Center).

Görgens-Albino, M., Mohammad, N., Blankhart, D. and Odutolu, O. (2007) *The Africa Multi-Country AIDS Program 2000–2006: Results of the World Bank's Response to a Development Crisis* (Washington DC: World Bank).

Grabowski (2002) 'Patents, Innovation and Access to New Pharmaceuticals', *Journal of International Economic Law*, 5(4): 849–60.

Green, E. C. (1992a) 'Sexually Transmitted Disease, Ethnomedicine and AIDS in Africa', *Social Science and Medicine*, 35(2): 121–30.

Green, E. C. (1992b) 'The Anthropology of Sexually Transmitted Disease in Liberia', *Social Science and Medicine*, 35(12): 1457–68.

Green, E. C. (1994) *AIDS and STDs in Africa* (Boulder: Westview Press).

Green, E. C. (2003) 'Culture Clash and AIDS Prevention', *The Responsive Community*, 13(4): 4–9.

Green, E. C. (2004) 'Indigenous Responses to AIDS in Africa', in 'Indigenous Knowledge: Local Pathways to Global Development', Report Marking Five Years of the World Bank Indigenous Knowledge for Development Programme, Knowledge and Learning Group, Africa Region.

Greyling, A. J. (2009) 'Reaching for the Dream: Quality Education for All', *Educational Studies*, 35(4): 425–35.

Guardian 27/09/2007.

Guardian 24/09/2009.

Hahn, B. H., Shaw, G. M., de Cock, K. M. and Sharp, P. M. (2000) 'AIDS as a Zoonosis: Scientific and Public Health Implications', *Science*, 287(5453): 607–14.

Hanefeld, J. (2009) 'The Role of Global Health Initiatives in Policy Implementation Processes Governing Antiretroviral Treatment (ART) Roll-out in Zambia and South Africa', Political Studies Association Annual Conference, Manchester, April.

Hanssen, K. N. (2005) 'Towards Multiparty System in Uganda: The Effect on Female Representation in Politics', Chr. Michelsen Institute, Working Paper, December.

Harris, B. (2004) 'Arranging Prejudice: Exploring Hate Crime in Post-Apartheid South Africa', Centre for the Study of Violence and Reconciliation Race and Citizenship in Transition Series.

Harris-Short, S. (2003) 'International Human Rights Law: Imperialist, Inept and Ineffective? Cultural Relativism and the UN Convention on the Rights of the Child', *Human Rights Quarterly*, 25: 130–81.

Hassim, S. (2009) 'Democracy's Shadows: Sexual Rights and Gender Politics in the Rape Trial of Jacob Zuma', *African Studies*, 68(1): 57–77.

Heald, S. (1995) 'The Power of Sex: Some Reflections on the Caldwells' "African Sexuality" Thesis', *Africa: Journal of the International African Institute*, 65(4): 489–505.

Hearst, N. and Chen, S. (2004) 'Condom Promotion for AIDS Prevention in the Developing World: Is It Working?', *Studies in Family Planning*, 35(1): 39–47.

Heimer, C. A. (2007) 'Old Inequalities, New Disease: HIV/AIDS in Sub-Saharan Africa', *Annual Review of Sociology*, 33: 551–77.

Herek, G. M., Capitanio, J. P. and Widaman, K. F. (2002) 'HIV-Related Stigma and Knowledge in the United States: Prevalence and Trends, 1991–1999', *American Journal of Public Health*, 92(3): 371–7.

Hertz, T. (2004) 'Have Minimum Wages Benefited South Africa's Domestic Service Workers?', Conference Paper, African Development and Poverty Reduction, 13–15 October, Somerset West, South Africa.

Heywood, M. (2004) 'The Price of Denial', *Interfund Development Update*, 5(3): 94–122.

Higgins, T. (2006) 'A Reflection on the Uses and Limits of Western Feminism in a Global Context', *Thomas Jefferson Law Review*, 28: 423–47.

Hilborn, R. and Liermann, M. (1998) 'Standing on the Shoulders of Giants: Learning from Experience in Fisheries', *Reviews in Fish Biology and Fisheries*, 8(3): 273–83.

Hirsh, M. (2003) *At War With Ourselves: Why America is Squandering Its Chance to Build a Better World* (Oxford: Oxford University Press).

Hogg, R. (2006) 'Life Expectancy with HIV', *Relay*, 2(3): 4–6.

Holmes, K. K., Levine, R. and Weaver, M. (2004) 'Effectiveness of Condoms in Preventing Sexually Transmitted Infections', *Bulletin of the World Health Organisation*, 82(6): 454–61.

Home Office (2005) 'Angola: Country Report', Country Information and Policy Unit, Home Office, United Kingdom, April.

Homer-Dixon, T. F. (1994) 'Environmental Scarcities and Violent Conflict: Evidence from Cases', *International Security*, 19(1): 5–40.

Hooper, E. (1999) *The River: A Journey to the Source of HIV and AIDS* (London: Little Brown & Co).

Hope, R. (2007) 'Gender Equality and "Sugar Daddies": Cross-Generational Sex in the Time of HIV', MIDEGO Gender Equality Series, Technical Series Paper Number 3/07.

HRW (Human Rights Watch) (1995) 'South Africa: The State Response to Domestic Violence and Rape' <http://www.hrw.org/reports/1995/Safricawm-02.htm>.

HRW (1997) 'South Africa: Violence against Women and the Medico-Legal System' <http://www.hrw.org/reports/1997/safrica>.

HRW (2001) 'Scared at School: Violence against Girls in South African Schools' <http://www.hrw.org/reports/2001/safrica>.

HRW (2002) 'Ignorance Only: HIV/AIDS, Human Rights and Federally Funded Abstinence-Only Programs in the United States', Human Rights Watch, 14, 5(G).

HRW (2003) 'Just Die Quietly: Domestic Violence and Women's Vulnerability to HIV in Uganda', Human Rights Watch, 15, 15(A).

HRW (2004) 'Access to Condoms and HIV/AIDS Information: A Global Health and Human Rights Concern', Human Rights Watch Background Paper, December.

HRW (2005) 'The Less They Know the Better: Abstinence-Only HIV/AIDS Programs in Uganda', Human Rights Watch, 17, 4(A).

HRW (2007) 'Darfur 2007: Chaos by Design Peacekeeping Challenges for AMIS and UNAMID', Human Rights Watch, 19, 15(A).

HRW (2008) 'Five Years On: No Justice for Sexual Violence in Darfur', Human Rights Watch Report, April.

HRW (2009) 'Soldiers Who Rape, Commanders Who Condone Sexual Violence and Military Reform in the Democratic Republic of Congo', Human Rights Watch Report, July.

Hunt, C. W. (1989) 'Migrant Labor and Sexually Transmitted Disease: AIDS in Africa', *Journal of Health and Social Behavior*, 30(4): 353–73.

ICTJ (International Center for Transitional Justice) (2008) 'Backgrounder: Uganda', International Centre for Transitional Justice, June <http://www.ictj.org/static/Africa/Uganda/ICTJ_UGA_Backgrounder_wb2008.pdf>.

Ijsselmuiden, C. B., Steinberg, M. H., Padayachee, G. N., Schoub, B. D., Strauss, S. A. and Buch, E. (1988) 'AIDS and South Africa: Towards a Comprehensive Strategy (Part I) – The Worldwide Experience', *South African Medical Journal*, 73: 455–60.

Ikenberry, G. J. (2004) 'Illusions of Empire: Defining the New American Order', *Foreign Affairs*, March/April.

Iliffe, J. (1998) *East African Doctors* (Cambridge: Cambridge University Press).

Iliffe, J. (2004) *Honour in African History* (Cambridge: Cambridge University Press).

Iliffe, J. (2006) *The African AIDS Epidemic: A History* (Athens: Ohio University Press).

Ingstad, B. (1990) 'The Cultural Construction of AIDS and Its Consequences for Prevention in Botswana', *Medical Anthropology Quarterly*, 4(1): 28–40.

Inter-Parliamentary Union (2010) 'Women in National Parliaments', World Classification <http://www.ipu.org/wmn-e/classif.htm>.

Inyang, P. E. B. (1986) 'Ibibio Traditional Medicine – Theory, Practice, Training and Retrospect', *Pharmaceutical Biology*, 24(3): 134–46.

Ismail, A. M. (2005) 'Drug Lobby Second to None: How the Pharmaceutical Industry Gets Its Way in Washington', The Centre for Public Integrity, July 7 <http://www.publicintegrity.org>.

Jacobson, G. (2009) 'The 2008 Presidential and Congressional Elections: Anti-Bush Referendum and Prospects for the Democratic Majority', *Political Science Quarterly*, 124(1): 1–30.

Jewkes, R. K., Levin, J. and Penn-Kekana, L. (2002) 'Risk Factors for Domestic Violence: Findings from a South African Cross-Sectional Study', *Social Science and Medicine*, 55(9): 1603–17.

Jewkes, R. K., Levin, J. and Penn-Kekana, L. (2003) 'Gender Inequalities, Intimate Partner Violence and HIV Preventive Practices: Findings of a South African Cross-Sectional Study', *Social Science and Medicine*, 56(1): 125–34.

Jewkes, R. K., Sikweyiya, Y., Morrell, R. and Dunkle, K. (2009a) 'Understanding Men's Health and Use of Violence: Interface of Rape and HIV in South Africa', Medical Research Council Report, June.

Jewkes, R. K., Abrahams, N., Mathews, S., Seedat, M., Van Niekerk, A., Suffla, S. and Ratele, K. (2009b) 'Preventing Rape and Violence in South Africa: Call for Leadership in a New Agenda for Action', Medical Research Council, Policy Brief.

Jochelson, K. (1991) 'Human Immunodeficiency Virus and Migrant Labor in South Africa', *International Journal of Health Services*, 21(1): 157–73.

Jochelson, K. (1999) 'Sexually Transmitted Diseases in Nineteenth- and Early Twentieth-Century South Africa', in Setel, P. W., Lewis, M. and Lyons, M. (eds) *Histories of Sexually Transmitted Diseases and HIV/AIDS in Sub-Saharan Africa* (Westport: Greenwood Press), pp. 217–44.

Johnson, C. (1997) 'Is HIV the Cause of AIDS? An Interview with Eleni Papadopulos-Eleopulos', *Continuum*, Autumn <http://www.theperthgroup.com/INTERVIEWS/cjepe.html>.

Johnson, C. A. (2007) *Off the Map: How HIV/AIDS Programming is Failing Same-Sex Practicing People in Africa* (New York: The International Gay and Lesbian Human Rights Commission).

Johnson, K. E. (2002) 'AIDS as a US National Security Threat: Media Effects and Geographical Imaginations', *Feminist Media Studies*, 2(1): 81–96.

Johnson, R. W. (2009) *South Africa's Brave New World: The Beloved Country since the End of Apartheid* (London: Allen Lane).

Joubert, P. H. (1990) 'Poisoning Admissions of Black South Africans', *Clinical Toxicology*, 28(1): 85–94.

Kagan, J. (2009) 'On the State of Scholarship in the American Academy, and on the State of Humanity', *Rorotoko*, 18 September.

Kaiser Family Foundation (2005a) 'Many Teens Who Take "Virginity Pledges" Substitute Other High-Risk Behaviour for Intercourse, Study Says', Daily Report, 21 March.

Kaiser Family Foundation (2005b) 'The HIV/AIDS Epidemic in Botswana', Fact Sheet, October.

Kaiser Family Foundation (2005c) 'The HIV/AIDS Epidemic in Namibia', Fact Sheet, October.

Kaiser Family Foundation (2005d) 'The HIV/AIDS Epidemic in Zimbabwe', Fact Sheet, October.

Kale, R. (1995) 'South Africa's Health: Traditional Healers in South Africa – A Parallel Health Care System', *British Medical Journal*, 310: 1182–5.

Kalichman, S. C. (2009) *Denying AID: Conspiracy Theories, Pseudoscience, and Human Tragedy* (New York: Copernicus Books).

Kapur, R. (2002) 'The Tragedy of Victimisation Rhetoric: Resurrecting the "Native" Subject in International/Post-Colonial Feminist Legal Politics', *Harvard Human Rights Journal*, 15(1): 1–37.

Kark, S. L. (2003) 'The Social Pathology of Syphilis in Africans', *International Journal of Epidemiology*, 32(2): 181–6.

Kategekwa, J. (2009) 'Empty Promises: What Happened to "Development" in the WTO's Doha Round?', Oxfam Briefing Paper, Number 131, 16 July.

Kaufman, N. H. and Lindquist, S. A. (1995) 'Critiquing Gender-Neutral Treaty Language: The Convention on the Elimination of All Forms of Discrimination against Women', in Peters, J. and Wolper, A. (eds) *Women's Rights Human Rights* (London: Routledge), pp. 114–25.

Kay, J. F. and Jackson, A. (2008) 'Sex, Lies and Stereotypes: How Abstinence-Only Programs Harm Women and Girls', Legal Momentum and the Harvard Law School Human Rights Program and the Program on International Health and Human Rights, Booklet.

Keehn, E. N. (2009) 'The Equality Courts as a Tool for Gender Transformation', Sonke Gender Justice Network Report <http://www.ngopulse.org/files/resources/sonke_equality_court_case_study_2 009.pdf>.

Kennedy, D. (2002) 'The International Human Rights Movement: Part of the Problem?', *Harvard Human Rights Journal*, 15(1): 101–25.

Kesby, M., Fenton, K., Boylea, P. and Power, R. (2003) 'An Agenda for Future Research on HIV and Sexual Behaviour among African Migrant Communities in the UK', *Social Science and Medicine*, 57(9): 1573–92.

Keuth, H. (2005) *The Philosophy of Karl Popper* (Cambridge: Cambridge University Press).

Korber, B., Muldoon, M., Theiler, J., Gao, F., Gupta, R., Lapedes, A., Hahn, B. H., Wolinsky, S. and Bhattacharya, T. (2000) 'Timing the Ancestor of the HIV-1 Pandemic Strains', *Science*, 288(5472): 1789–96.

Kripke, G. and Weinberg, S. (2006) 'Public Health at Risk: A US Free Trade Agreement Could Threaten Access to Medicines in Thailand', Oxfam Briefing Paper, Number 86, April.

Krishnadas, J. (2006) 'The Sexual Subaltern in Conversations "Somewhere in Between": Law and the Old Politics of Colonialism', *Feminist Legal Studies*, 14: 53–77.

Kyle, W. S. (1992) 'Simian Retroviruses, Polio Vaccine, and Origin of AIDS', *Lancet*, 339(8793): 600–1.

Lambkin, F. J. (1914) 'An Outbreak of Syphilis on a Virgin Soil: Notes on Syphilis in the Uganda Protectorate', in Power, D. A. and Murphy, K. (eds) *A System of Syphilis*, Volume 2 (London): 339–55.

Le Blanc, M., Meintel, D. and Piché, V. (1991) 'The African Sexual System: Comment on Caldwell et al', *Population and Development Review*, 17(3): 497–505.

Leggett, T. (2003) 'The Sieve Effect South Africa's Conviction Rates in Perspective', Institute for Security Studies Paper, September.

Lewis, S. (2002) 'Statement by Stephen Lewis, the Secretary-General's UN Envoy on HIV/AIDS in Africa', Noon Briefing of UN Media, 3 July.

Liddell, C., Barrett, L. and Bydawell, M. (2005) 'Indigenous Representations of Illness and AIDS in Sub-Saharan Africa', *Social Science and Medicine*, 60(4): 691–700.

Liversidge, A. F. (1995) 'The Limits of Science: In Science, as in Life, Truth is Not Always Value-Free – A Case Study in Careerist Politics', *The Cultural Studies Times*, Fall <http://www.virusmyth.com/aids/hiv/allimits.htm>.

Liversidge, A. F. (2001) 'The Scorn of Heretics', Conference on Science and Democracy, Naples, April.

Lòpez Trujillo, A. (2003) 'Family Values versus Safe Sex – A Reflection by His Eminence', Pontifical Council for the Family, December.

Love, J. (2002) 'Access to Medicine and Compliance with the WTO TRIPS Accord: Models for State Practise in Developing Countries', in Drahos, P. and Mayne, R. (eds) *Global Intellectual Property Rights: Knowledge, Access and Development* (Basingstoke: Palgrave Macmillan), pp. 74–89.

Lowi, M. (1992) 'West Bank Water Resources and the Resolution of Conflict in the Middle East', Project on Environmental Change and Acute Conflict, Trudeau Centre for Peace and Conflict Studies, University of Toronto, Occasional Paper Series, Occasional Paper, Number 1, September.

Lozano Barragán, J. (2006) 'Statement by Javier Lozano Barragán: Permanent Observer Mission of the Holy See to the United Nations', 2 June.

Luke, N. and Kurz, K. M. (2002) 'Cross-generational and Transactional Sexual Relations in Sub-Saharan Africa: Prevalence of Behavior and Implications for Negotiating Safer Sexual Practices', International Centre for Research on Women, September.

Lwanda, J. L. (2003) 'Politics, Culture and Medicine: An Unholy Trinity? Historical Continuities and Ruptures in the HIV/AIDS Story in Malawi', in Kalipeni, E., Craddock, S., Oppong, J. R. and Ghosh, J. (eds) *HIV and AIDS in Africa: Beyond Epidemiology* (Oxford: Wiley-Blackwell), pp. 29–44.

Lyons, A. P. and Lyons, H. D. (2004) *Irregular Connections: A History of Anthropology and Sexuality* (Lincoln: University of Nebraska Press).

Maddox, J. (1993) 'Has Duesberg a Right of Reply?', *Nature*, 363(6425): 109.

Mail and Guardian 18/10/2004.

Mail and Guardian 12/06/2006.

Mail and Guardian 24/02/2008.

Makgoba, M. W., Solomon, N. and Tucker, T. J. P. (2002) 'Science, Medicine, and the Future: The Search for an HIV Vaccine', *British Medical Journal*, 324: 211–13.

Malowany, M. (2000) 'Unfinished Agendas: Writing the History of Medicine of Sub-Saharan Africa', *African Affairs*, 99(395): 325–49.

Mann, C. C. (2005) *1491: New Revelations of the Americas Before Columbus* (New York: Vintage).

Marks, S. (2002) 'An Epidemic Waiting to Happen? The Spread of HIV/AIDS in South Africa in Social and Historical Perspective', *African Studies*, 61(1): 13–26.

Marks, S. and Andersson, N. (1990) 'The Epidemiology and Culture of Violence', in Chabani Manganyi, N. and du Toit, A. (eds) *Political Violence and the Struggle in South Africa* (Basingstoke: Macmillan), pp. 29–69.

Martin, B. (2001) 'The Burden of Proof and the Origin of Acquired Immune Deficiency Syndrome', *The Royal Society, Philosophical Transactions B*, 356(1410): 939–44.

Marx, P., Alcabes, P. and Drucker, E. (2001) 'Serial Human Passage of Simian Immunodeficiency Virus by Unsterile Injections and the Emergence of Epidemic Human Immunodeficiency Virus in Africa', *The Royal Society, Philosophical Transactions B*, 356(1410): 911–20.

Marx, P. A. (2005) 'Unsolved Questions Over the Origin of HIV and AIDS', *American Society for Microbiology News*, 71(1): 15–20.

Mayne, R. (2002a) 'The Global Campaign on Patents and Access to Medicines: An Oxfam Perspective', in Drahos, P. and Mayne, R. (eds) *Global Intellectual Property Rights: Knowledge, Access and Development* (Basingstoke: Palgrave Macmillan), pp. 244–58.

Mayne, R. (2002b) 'US Bullying on Drug Patents: One Year after Doha', Oxfam Briefing Paper, Number 33, November.

Mayne, R. (2005) 'Regionalism, Bilateralism, and "TRIP Plus" Agreements: The Threat to Developing Countries', Human Development Report Office Occasional Paper, November.

Mbeki, T. (2000a) 'Letter to World Leaders', *Sunday Times*, 3 April.

Mbeki, T. (2000b) 'Speech of the President of South Africa at the Opening Session of the Conference', XIII International AIDS Conference, Durban, South Africa.

Mbeki, T. (2004) 'When is Good News Bad News?', *ANC Today*, 4(39), 1–7 October <http://www.anc.org.za/ancdocs/anctoday/2004/at39.htm>.

McI, T. F. (1921) 'Review: *The Ilai Speaking Peoples of Northern Rhodesia* by Rev. E. W. Smith and Captain A. M. Dale', *Journal of the African Society*, 78: 150–2.

McClintock, A. (1995) *Imperial Leather: Race, Gender and Sexuality in the Colonial Contest* (London: Routledge).

McCormack, G. P., Glynn, J. R., Crampin, A. C., Sibande, F., Mulawa, D., Bliss, L., Broadbent, P., Abarca, K., Ponninghaus, J. M., Fine, P. E. M. and Clewley, J. P. (2002) 'Early Evolution of the Human Immunodeficiency Virus Type 1, Subtype C Epidemic in Rural Malawi', *Journal of Virology*, 76(24): 12890–9.

Mdhluli, M., Seier, J. V., Dhansay, M. A. and Laubscher, A. J. (2004) 'A Toxicity Study of LEAF Consumption', Report for the Medical Research Council of South Africa, August.

Meekersa, D. and Calvès, A. E. (1997) '"Main" Girlfriends, Girlfriends, Marriage, and Money: The Social Context of HIV Risk Behaviour in Sub-Saharan Africa', *Health Transition Review*, Supplement to Volume 7: 361–75.

Meredith, M. (2006a) *The State of Africa: A History of Fifty Years of Independence* (London: Free).

Meredith, M. (2006b) *The Fate of Africa: From the Hopes of Freedom to the Heart of Despair – A History of Fifty Years of Independence* (New York: Public Affairs).

Meyer-Weitz, A., Reddy, P., Weijts, W., van den Borne, B. and Kok, G. (1998) 'The Socio-Cultural Contexts of Sexually Transmitted Diseases in South Africa: Implications for Health Education Programmes', *AIDS Care*, 10 (Supp 1): S39–55.

Miguel, E. (2004) 'Poverty and Witch Killing', *Review of Economic Studies*, 72(4): 1153–72.

Mill, J. S. (1998) *On Liberty and Other Essays* (Oxford: Oxford University Press).

Mills, E. (2006) 'HIV Illness Meanings and Collaborative Healing Strategies in South Africa', CSSR Working Paper, Number 157, May <http://www.cssr.uct.ac.za/sites/cssr.uct.ac.za/files/pubs/wp157.pdf>.

Mills, E., Cooper, C., Seely, D. and Kanfer, I. (2005) 'African Herbal Medicines in the Treatment of HIV: Hypoxis and Sutherlandia. An Overview of Evidence and Pharmacology', *Nutrition Journal*, 4(19).

MMM (Medical Missionaries of Mary) (2008) *Healing and Development: Yearbook of the Medical Missionaries of Mary* (Dublin: MMM Communications).

Moffett, H. (2006) '"These Women, They Force Us to Rape Them": Rape as Narrative of Social Control in Post-Apartheid South Africa', *Journal of Southern African Studies*, 32(1): 129–44.

Mohanty, C. T. (1991) 'Under Western Eyes: Feminist Scholarship and Colonial Discourses', in Mohanty, C., Russo, A. and Torres, L. (eds) *Third World Women and the Politics of Feminism* (Indiana: Indiana University Press), pp. 334–53.

Morgan, L. (2009) 'What's on the Agenda in Global Health? The Experts' List for the Obama Administration', Centre for Global Development Notes, June.

Moore, J. (2004) 'The Puzzling Origin of AIDS', *American Scientist*, 92: 540–7.

Moore, J. (2006) 'HIV Science and Responsible Journalism', XVI International AIDS Conference, Toronto.

MSF (Médecins Sans Frontières) (2007) 'The Second-Line AIDS Crisis: Condemned to Repeat?', Médecins Sans Frontières, Field News, 11 April <http://doctorswithoutborders.org/news/article.cfm?id=3488&cat=field-news>.

MSF (2009) 'Need for Newer Drugs', Médecins Sans Frontières, July <http://www.msfaccess.org/main/hiv-aids/introduction-to-hivaids/need-for-newer-drugs/>.

MSF (2010) 'Experience Treating the Most Neglected of the Neglected Tropical Diseases (NTDs)', Médecins Sans Frontières (MSF) Report.

Mullis, K. (1998) *Dancing Naked in the Mind Field* (New York: Vintage).

Murray, L. and Burnham, G. (2009) 'Understanding Childhood Sexual Abuse in Africa', *Lancet*, 373(9679): 1924–6.

Museveni, J. K. (2004) 'Common Ground: A Shared Vision for Health', The Medical Institute for Sexual Health, Washington DC.

Museveni, Y. (2000) 'Statement by the President of Uganda', Paper Presented at the African Development Forum, Addis Ababa.

Museveni, Y. (2004) Report by H.E Yoweri Kaguta Museveni, President of the Republic of Uganda, XIV International Conference on AIDS and STDs on Political Commitment and Accountability, Bangkok.

Museveni, Y. (2008) 'Opening Ceremony', PEPFAR; the Global Fund to Fight AIDS, Tuberculosis and Malaria; UNAIDS; UNICEF; the World Bank and the

World Health Organization, 3 June <http://www.kaisernetwork.org/health_cast/uploaded_files/060308_hivimplementers_opening_transcript.pdf>.

Nakkazi, E. (2006) 'Uganda: HIV Patients Die as ARVs Expire', *Africa News Update*, 9 September <http://www.afrika.no/Detailed/12763.html>.

National Academy of Public Administration (2006) 'Mitigating HIV/AIDS' Impacts on Teachers and Administrators in Sub-Saharan Africa', Academy International Affairs Working Paper Series <http://www.napawash.org/Pubs/africa.pdf>.

National Institute for Health Care Management (2002) 'Changing Patterns of Pharmaceutical Innovation', Research Report, May.

National Intelligence Council (2000) 'The Global Infectious Disease Threat and its Implications for the United States', NIE 99-17D, January.

Nattrass, N. (2006) 'AIDS, Science and Governance: The Battle Over Antiretroviral Therapy in Post-Apartheid South Africa', Centre for Social Science Research, University of Cape Town.

Nattrass, N. (2007) 'AIDS: Denialism vs Science', *Skeptical Enquirer*, 31(5).

Nattrass, N. (2008) 'AIDS and the Scientific Governance of Medicine in Post-Apartheid South Africa', *African Affairs*, 107(427): 157–76.

Nattrass, N. (2010) 'Still Crazy After All These Years: The Challenge of AIDS Denialism for Science', *AIDS and Behavior*, 14(2): 248–51.

Nel, J. A. and Judge, M. (2008) 'Exploring Homophobic Victimisation in Gauteng, South Africa: Issues, Impact and Responses', *Acta Criminologica*, 21(3): 19–36.

New Scientist 30/09/2006.

New Vision 20/04/2005.

New Vision 14/07/2008.

Ngcobo, M. (2007) 'Doctors For Life Accused of Sabotaging Traditional Healers', *Health-e Bulletin*, 25 June.

Ngubane, H. (1977) *Body and Mind in Zulu Medicine* (London: Academic Press).

Nguyen, V. K. and Stovel, K. (2004) 'The Social Science of HIV/AIDS: A Critical Review and a Priorities for Action', Social Science Research Council Working Group on HIV/AIDS, October.

NIAID (National Institute of Allergy and Infectious Diseases) (2009) 'HIV Vaccine Regimen Demonstrates Modest Preventive Effect in Thailand Clinical Study', National Institute of Allergy and Infectious Diseases (NIAID) Press Release, 24 September.

Niehaus, I. (2001) *Witchcraft, Power and Politics: Exploring the Occult in the South African Lowveld* (London: Pluto Press).

Ntloedibe-Kuswani, G. (1999) 'Bongaka, Women and Witchcraft', Women's Worlds 99: The 7th International Interdisciplinary Congress on Women, Session VII: Gendering the Past, Norway.

Nujoma, S. (2000) 'Address by His Excellency Mr Sam Nujoma, President of the Republic of Namibia', 88th Session of the International Labour Organisation Conference, Geneva, Thursday, 8 June.

Obama, B. (2008) 'Barack Obama: Fighting HIV/AIDS Worldwide', Obama 2008 <http://www.barackobama.com/pdf/AIDSFactSheet.pdf>.

Odebiyi, A. and Vivekananda, F. (1991) 'AIDS in Third World Countries: Africa What are the Alternatives', *Scandinavian Journal of Development Alternatives*, X(1&2): 91–9.

OECD (2009) 'Measuring Aid to HIV/AIDS Control', Updated Statistics on Aid to HIV/AIDS Control, April.

OECD (2010) 'Development Aid at a Glance 2010: Statistics by Region', Aid Statistics.

Ojo, O. (1990) 'Understanding Human Rights in Africa', in Bertin, J., Baehr, P. R., Burger, J. H., Flinterman, C., de Klerk, B., Kroes, R., van Minnen, C. A. and Van der Wal, K. (eds) *Human Rights in a Pluralist World: Individuals and Collectivities* (Westport and London: Meckler): 115–23.

Okpako, D. T. (1999) 'Traditional African Medicine: Theory and Pharmacology Explored', *Trends in Pharmacological Sciences*, 20(12): 482–5.

Onyejekwe, C. J. (2004) 'The Interrelationship Between Gender-based Violence and HIV/AIDS in South Africa', *Journal of International Women's Studies*, 6(1): 34–40.

Oomman, N., Bernstein, M. and Rosenzweig, S. (2007) 'Following the Funding for HIV/AIDS: A Comparative Analysis of the Funding Practices of PEPFAR, the Global Fund and World Bank MAP in Mozambique, Uganda and Zambia', Center for Global Development – HIV/AIDS Monitor Tracking Aid Effectiveness, 10 October.

Oomman, N., Bernstein, M. and Rosenzweig, S. (2008) 'The Numbers Behind the Stories: PEPFAR Funding for Fiscal Years 2004 to 2006', Centre for Global Development.

Oppong, C. (1973) 'Notes on Cultural Aspects of Menstruation in Ghana', *Institute of African Studies Research Review*, IX(2): 33–8.

Oppong, J. R. and Agyei-Mensah, S. (2003) 'AIDS in West Africa: The Case of Senegal, Ghana and Nigeria', in Kalipeni, E., Craddock, S., Oppong, J. R. and Ghosh, J. (eds) *HIV and AIDS in Africa: Beyond Epidemiology* (Oxford: Wiley-Blackwell).

Orubuloye, I. O. and Oguntimehin, F. (1999) 'Death is Pre-Ordained, It Will Come When It Is Due: Attitudes of Men to Death in the Presence of AIDS in Nigeria', in Caldwell, J. C., Caldwell, P., Anarfi, J., Awusabo-Asare, K., Ntozi, J., Orubuloye, I. O., Marck, J., Cosford, W., Colombo, R. and Hollings, E. (eds) *Resistances to Behavioural Change to Reduce HIV/AIDS Infection in Predominantly Heterosexual Epidemics in Third World Countries* (Canberra: Australian National University), pp. 101–11.

Osoba, A. O. (1981) 'Sexually Transmitted Diseases in Tropical Africa: A Review of the Present Situation', *British Journal of Venereal Disease*, 57(2): 89–94.

Osterhaus, A. (2001) 'Catastrophes after Crossing Species Barriers', *The Royal Society, Philosophical Transactions B*, 356(1410): 791–3.

Outwater, A., Abrahams, N. and Campbell, J. C. (2005) 'Women in South Africa: Intentional Violence and HIV/AIDS – Intersections and Prevention', *Journal of Black Studies*, 35(4): 135–54.

Packard, R. M. and Epstein, P. (1991) 'Epidemiologists, Social Scientists, and the Structure of Medical Research on AIDS in Africa', *Social Science and Medicine*, 33(7): 771–93.

Pakenham, T. (1992) *The Scramble for Africa* (London: Abacas).

Papadopulos-Eleopulos, E. (2006) 'Response to Professor John Moore by the Perth Group', Open Letter, 23 September.

Parikh, S. (2007) 'The Political Economy of Marriage and HIV: The ABC Approach, "Safe" Infidelity, and Managing Moral Risk in Uganda', *American Journal of Public Health*, 97(7): 1198–208.

Paroske, M. (2009) 'Deliberating International Science Policy Controversies: Uncertainty and AIDS in South Africa', *Quarterly Journal of Speech*, 95(2): 148–70.

Pascal, L. (1991) 'What Happens When Science Goes Bad? The Corruption of Science and the Origins of AIDS: A Study in Spontaneous Generation', University of Wollongong, Working Paper.

Patterson, A. S. (2006) *The Politics of AIDS in Africa* (Boulder: Lynne Reiner).

Peacock, D. and Levack, A. (2004) 'The Men as Partners Program in South Africa: Reaching Men to End Gender-Based Violence and Promote Sexual and Reproductive Health', *International Journal of Men's Health*, 3(3): 173–88.

Pekala, A. Z. D. (2007) 'Traditional Medicines and HIV/AIDS', *Medical Journal of Therapeutics Africa*, 1(2): 94–5.

Peltzer, K., Nqeketo, A., Petros, G. and Kanta, X. (2008) 'Traditional Circumcision During Manhood Initiation Rituals in the Eastern Cape, South Africa: A Pre-Post Intervention Evaluation', BMC Public Health, 8(64) <http://www.biomedcentral.com/content/pdf/1471-2458-8-64.pdf>.

PEPFAR (2005) 'Defining the ABC Approach', Guidance for PEPFAR Partnership Frameworks and Partnership Framework Implementation Plans <http://www.pepfar.gov/guidance/75837.htm>.

PEPFAR (2008) 'The Power of Partnerships: The U.S. President's Emergency Plan for AIDS Relief', 2008 Annual Report to Congress <http://www.pepfar.gov/documents/organization/100029.pdf>.

PEPFAR (2009a) 'The U.S. Commitment to Global HIV/AIDS', PEPFAR Overview, January Update <http://www.pepfar.gov/press/81352.htm>.

PEPFAR (2009b) 'Comprehensive Country-Specific Information about PEPFAR-Supported Efforts' <http://www.pepfar.gov/countries>.

PEPFAR (2009c) 'Celebrating Life: The U.S. President's Emergency Plan for AIDS Relief', 2009 Annual Report to Congress.

PEPFAR (2010) 'Making a Difference: Funding', Fact Sheet, March <http://www.pepfar.gov/documents/organization/80161.pdf>.

Pettman, J. J. (1996) *Worlding Women: A Feminist International Politics* (London: Routledge).

PhRMA (2007) 'Drug Discovery and Development: Understanding the R&D Process', Pharmaceutical Research and Manufacturers of America, February.

PhRMA (2010) 'Who We Are', Pharmaceutical Research and Manufacturers of America <http://www.phrma.org/about_phrma>.

Picciotto, S. (2002) 'Defending the Public Interest in TRIPS and the WTO', in Drahos, P. and Mayne, R. (eds) *Global Intellectual Property Rights: Knowledge, Access and Development* (Basingstoke: Palgrave Macmillan), pp. 224–43.

Pick, D. (1993) *Faces of Degeneration: A European Disorder c.1848–c.1918* (Cambridge: Cambridge University Press).

Pickup, F. (2001) *Ending Violence against Women: A Challenge for Development and Humanitarian Work* (Oxford: Oxfam).

Pijper, A. (1919) 'Damaged Goods', *South African Medical Record*, 17, 8 November, pp. 323–5.

Pontifical Council for the Family (1996) *The Truth and Meaning of Human Sexuality: Guidelines for Education within the Family* (Rome: Vatican).

Popat, A., Shear, N. H., Malkiewicz, I., Stewartc, M. J., Steenkamp, V., Thomson, S. and Neuman, M. G. (2001) 'The Toxicity of Callilepis Laureola, a South African Traditional Herbal Medicine', *Clinical Biochemistry*, 34(3): 229–36.

Prakash, S. (2005) 'Tanga AIDS Working Group: Case Study', World Bank Note, Integration of Local Knowledge into the Multi-Country AIDS Programs <http://www.worldbank.org/afr/ik/dlc/aids/Tawg.pdf>.

Prendergast, J. and Norris, J. (2009) 'Obama, Africa and Peace', Enough Strategy Paper, 13 January.

Puckett, L. A. and Reynolds, W. L. (1996) 'Rules, Sanctions and Enforcement Under Section 301: At Odds with the WTO?', *American Journal of International Law*, 90(4): 675–89.

Putzel, J. (2004) 'The Politics of Action on AIDS: A Case Study of Uganda', *Public Administration and Development*, 24(1): 19–30.

Radelet, S., Schutte, R. and Abarcar, P. (2008) 'What's Behind the Recent Declines in US Foreign Assistance?', Center for Global Development, December.

Rampen, F. (1978) 'Venereal Syphilis in Tropical Africa', *British Journal of Venereal Diseases*, 54(6): 364–8.

RAPCAN (2008) 'Crimes Against Children', Fact Sheet <http://www.rapcan.org.za/File_uploads/Resources/Fact%20Sheet%20Violen ce%20against%20Children% 202008.pdf>.

RED (2010) '$140 Million Contributed to the Global Fund', Impact <http://www.joinred.com/#impact>.

Reinikka, R. and Svensson, J. (2003) 'Working for God? Evaluating Service Delivery of Religious Not-for-Profit Health Care Providers in Uganda', World Bank Research Working Paper, Number 3058.

Revkin, A. C. (2009) 'Skeptics Dispute Climate Worries and Each Other', *New York Times*, 8 March.

Richards, T. (2006) 'The Great Medicines Scandal', *British Medical Journal*, 332(7554): 1345–6.

Robins, S. (2008) 'Sexual Politics and the Zuma Rape Trial', *Journal of Southern African Studies*, 34(2): 411–27.

Rödlach, A. (2006) *Witches, Westerners and HIV: AIDS and Cultures of Blame in Africa* (Walnut Creek: Left Coast Press).

Romero-Daza, N. (2002) 'Traditional Medicine in Africa', *The ANNALS of the American Academy of Political and Social Science*, 583: 173–6.

Ryan, M. P. (1998) *Knowledge Diplomacy: Global Competition and the Politics of Intellectual Property* (Washington DC: Brookings Institution Press).

Samuel, M. C. and Engel, R. R. (1988) 'Selected Aspects of AIDS among Homosexual Men', *Social and Preventive Medicine*, 33(7): 331–5.

Sampath, P. G. (2005) 'Breaking the Fence: Can Patent Rights Deter Biomedical Innovation in "Technology Followers"?', United Nations University Discussion Paper Series, December 2005.

SAPS (2005) 'Crime Report 2005', South African Police Service <http://www.saps.gov.za/statistics/reports/crimestats/2005/_pdf/crimes/rape.pdf>.

SAPS (2009) 'Annual Report', South African Police Service.

Schneider, W. H. (2009) 'Smallpox in Africa during Colonial Rule', *Medical History*, 53(2): 193–227.

Schneider, W. H. and Drucker, E. (2006) 'Blood Transfusions in the Early Years of AIDS in Sub-Saharan Africa', *American Journal of Public Health*, 96(6): 984–94.

Schoepf, B. G. (2002) '"Mobutu's Disease": A Social History of AIDS in Kinshasa', *Review of African Political Economy*, 29(93/94): 561–73.

Schraeder, P. J. (2004) *African Politics and Society. A Mosaic in Transformation,* Second Edition (Belmont, CA: Thomson-Wadsworth).

Science 10/10/2008.

Scientific American 06/10/2008.

Seier, J. V., Mdhluli, M., Dhansay, M. A., Loza, J. and Laubscher, R. (2002) 'A Toxicity Study of Sutherlandia Leaf Powder (*Sutherlandia microphylla*) Consumption', Report for the Medical Research Council of South Africa and the National Research Foundation.

Seidel, R. (2005) 'Behavior Change Perspectives and Communication Guidelines on Six Child Survival Interventions', A Joint Publication of the Academy Educational Development and the John Hopkins Bloomberg School of Public Health.

Sell, S. K. (1995) 'Intellectual Property Protection and Antitrust in the Developing World: Crisis, Coercion, and Choice', *International Organization,* 49(2): 315–49.

Sell, S. K. (2007) 'TRIPS-Plus Free Trade Agreements and Access to Medicines', *Liverpool Law Review,* 28(1): 41–75.

Sharp, P. M., Bailes, E., Gao, F., Beer, B. E., Hirsch, V. M. and Hahn, B. H. (2000) 'Origins and Evolution of AIDS Viruses: Estimating the Timescale', *Biochemical Society Transactions,* 28(2): 275–82.

Shilts, R. (1987) *And the Band Played On: Politics, People and the AIDS Epidemic* (New York: Penguin).

Shinn, D. H. (2008) 'African Migration and the Brain Drain', Paper Presented at the Institute for African Studies and Slovenia Global Action, Ljubljana, Slovenia, 20 June.

Sidley, P. (2001) 'Drug Companies Sue South African Government over Generics', *British Medical Journal,* 322(7284): 447.

Silberschmidt, M. and Rasch, V. (2001) 'Adolescent Girls, Illegal Abortions and "Sugar Daddies" in Dar es Salaam: Vulnerable Victim and Active Social Agents', *Social Science and Medicine,* 52(12): 1815–26.

Singh, S., Darroch, J. E. and Bankole, A. (2003) 'A, B and C in Uganda: The Roles of Abstinence, Monogamy and Condom Use in HIV Decline', The Alan Guttmacher Institute, Occasional Report, Number 9.

Smith, A. M., Maher, J., Simmons, J. and Dolan, M. (2004) 'HIV Prevention from the Perspective of a Faith-Based Development Agency', CAFOD Paper.

Smith, E. W. and Dale, A. M. (2003) *Ila Speaking Peoples of Northern Rhodesia, Part 1* (Montana: Kessinger).

Smoak, N. D., Scott-Sheldon, L. A. J., Johnson, B. T., Carey, M. P. and SHARP Research Team (2006) 'Sexual Risk Reduction Interventions Do Not Inadvertently Increase the Overall Frequency of Sexual Behaviour: A Meta-Analysis of 174 Studies with 116,735 Participants', *Journal of Acquired Immune Deficiency Syndrome,* 41(3): 374–84.

Smyth, A. S. H. (2006) 'AIDS: Time to Stop Ignoring the Truth', *The First Post,* 27 December.

Spiegel, A. D. (1991) 'Polygyny as Myth: Towards Understanding Extramarital Relations in Lesotho', *African Studies,* 50(1–2): 145–66.

Ssenyonjo, M. (2007) 'Women's Rights to Equality and Non-discrimination: Discriminatory Family Legislation in Uganda and the Role of Uganda's Constitutional Court', *International Journal of Law, Policy and the Family,* 21(3): 341–72.

Steenkamp, V. (2002) 'Toxicology of Traditional Remedies', *Science in Africa*, February.

Steenkamp, V., Stewart, M. J., Curowska, E. and Zuckerman, M. (2002) 'A Severe Case of Multiple Metal Poisoning in a Child Treated with a Traditional Medicine', *Forensic Science International*, 128(3): 123–6.

Steinbrook, R. (2007) 'Thailand and the Compulsory Licensing of Efavirenz', *The New England Journal of Medicine*, 356(6): 544–6.

Stemmet, J. (2003) 'From Nipples and Nationalists to Full Frontal in the New South Africa: A Brief Introduction to the History of Pornography and the Censorship thereof in the Old and New South Africa', Biennial Conference of the South African Historical Society, University of the Free State, 29 June–1 July.

Stewart, M. J., Moar, J. J., Steenkamp, P. and Kokot, M. (1999) 'Findings in Fatal Cases of Poisoning Attributed to Traditional Remedies in South Africa', *Forensic Science International*, 101(3): 177–83.

Stobart, E. (2006) 'Child Abuse Linked to Accusations of "Possession" and "Witch-craft"', Department for Education and Skills (UK) Research Paper, Number 750.

Stock, R. (1981) 'Traditional Healers in Rural Hausaland', *GeoJournal*, 5(4): 363–8.

Stoler, A. L. (1989) 'Making Empire Respectable: The Politics of Race and Sexual Morality in 20th-Century Colonial Cultures', *American Ethnologist*, 16(4): 634–60.

South African Government (1996a) 'National Drug Policy', Department of Health, January <http://www.doh.gov.za/docs/policy/drugsjan1996.pdf>.

South African Government (1996b) 'Constitution of the Republic of South Africa' <http://www.info.gov.za/documents/constitution/1996/96cons.htm#39>.

South African Government (1998) 'Republic of South Africa Domestic Violence Act' <http://www.info.gov.za/view/DownloadFileAction?id=70651>.

South African Government (2003) 'The Traditional Health Practitioners Act' <http://www.doh.gov.za/docs/bills/thb.html>.

South African Government (2007) 'The Violent Nature of Crime in South Africa', A Concept Paper for the Justice, Crime Prevention and Security Cluster, Department of Safety and Security, 25 June.

Suhrke, A. (1993) 'Pressure Points: Environmental Degradation, Migration and Conflict', Project on Environmental Change and Acute Conflict, Trudeau Centre for Peace and Conflict Studies, University of Toronto, Occasional Paper Series, Number 3, March.

Supreme Court of South Australia (2007) R v Parenzee, SACS 143, Reasons for Decision of The Honourable Justice Sulan, 27 April.

Susser, I. (2009) *AIDS, Sex, and Culture: Global Politics and Survival in Southern Africa* (Chichester: Wiley-Blackwell).

Sweeney, A. W. (1999) 'Editorial – Prospects for Control of Mosquito-Borne Diseases', *Journal of Medical Microbiology*, 48: 879–81.

Tabe, A. (2006) 'Poverty Blamed for Africa's Lack of Access to Cheap Anti-retrovirals', Voice of America, 6 December <http://www.aegis.com/news/voa/2006/VA06-1210.html>.

TAC (2008) 'Translation of Ubhejane Video Transcript Received from Thandiwe', Transcript <http://www.tac.org.za/community/files/TranslationOfUbhejaneVideo-Transcript.pdf>.

Tagwireyi, D., Ball, D. E. and Nhachi, C. F. B. (2002) 'Traditional Medicine Poisoning in Zimbabwe: Clinical Presentation and Management in Adults', *Human & Experimental Toxicology*, 21(11): 579–86.

Taubenberger, J. K. and Morens, D. M. (2006) '1918 Influenza: The Mother of All Pandemics', *Emerging Infectious Diseases*, 12(1): 15–22.

The Lancet (2009) 'Redemption for the Pope?', Editorial, 373(9669), March: 1054.

Thomas, F. (2008) 'Indigenous Narratives of HIV/AIDS: Morality and Blame in a Time of Change', *Medical Anthropology*, 27(3): 227–56.

Thomas, J. R. (2001) 'HIV/AIDS Drugs, Patents and the TRIPS Agreement: Issues and Options', CRS Report for Congress, 27 July.

Thomson, A. (2010) *An Introduction to African Politics*, Third Edition (London: Routledge).

Torday, E. (1929) 'The Principles of Bantu Marriage', *Africa: Journal of the International African Institute*, 2(3): 255–90.

Tordoff, W. (2002) *Government and Politics in Africa*, Fourth Edition (Basingstoke: Macmillan).

Trenholm, C., Devaney, B., Fortson, K., Quay, L., Wheeler, J. and Clark, M. (2007) 'Impacts of Four Title V, Section 510 Abstinence Education Programs – Final Report', Mathematica Policy Research.

Tshabalala-Msimang, M. (2004) 'Speech by the Minister of Health at the Launch of the Kokosi "Rudo" Home based Care', Carltonville, 8 October.

Tshabalala-Msimang, M. (2007) 'Speech by Health Minister Manto Tshabalala-Msimang on African Traditional Medicine Day', Department of Health, 6 September.

Tumushabe, J. (2006) 'The Politics of HIV/AIDS in Uganda', United Nations Research Institute for Social Policy, Programme Paper Number 28.

Tyfield, D. (2008) 'Enabling TRIPs: The Pharma–Biotech–University Patent Coalition', *Review of International Political Economy*, 15(4): 535–66.

Ugandan Government (2006) 'Uganda HIV/AIDS Sero-Behavioural Survey 2004–2005', Ministry of Health.

Ugandan Government (2008) 'UNGASS Country Progress Report: Uganda', Period January 2006 to December 2007, Uganda AIDS Commission, January.

UN (1992) Declaration on the Elimination of Violence against Women, A/RES/48/104 <http://www.unhchr.ch/huridocda/huridoca.nsf/(Symbol)/A.RES.48.104.En>.

UN (1993a) 'Vienna Declaration and Programme of Action', A/CONF.157/23 <http://www.unhchr.ch/huridocda/huridoca.nsf/(Symbol)/ACONF157.23.En>.

UN (1993b) 'Declaration on the Elimination of Violence against Women', A/RES/48/104 <http://www.unhchr.ch/huridocda/huridoca.nsf/(symbol)/a.res.48.104.en>.

UN (1995) Report of the Fourth World Conference on Women, Beijing, 4–15 September, A/CONF.177/20/Rev.1 <http://www.un.org/womenwatch/daw/beijing/pdf/Beijing%20full%20report%20E.pdf>.

UN (2000) 'Security Council Holds Debate on Impact of AIDS on Peace and Security in Africa', Press Release, UNIS/SC/1173, 11 January.

UN (2001) 'Declaration of Commitment on HIV/AIDS', United Nations General Assembly Special Session on HIV/AIDS, 25–27 June.

UN (2003) 'Strategic Programme Framework on Crime and Drugs for Southern Africa', Report by the United Nations Office on Drugs and Crime.

UN (2004) *The Impact of AIDS* (New York: United Nations).

UN (2006a) 'Declaration of Commitment on HIV/AIDS', United Nations General Assembly Special Session on HIV/AIDS, 31 May–1 June.

UN (2006b) 'Responses to the List of Issues and Questions for Consideration of the Combined Third, Fourth and Fifth Periodic Report', Committee on the Elimination of Discrimination against Women Pre-Session Working Group, Thirty-sixth session, 7–25 August.

UN (2010) 'Updated Comprehensive Framework for Action', High Level Task Force on the Global Food Crisis, Dublin Draft, 10 May.

UNAIDS (2000a) 'Evaluation of the 100% Condom Programme in Thailand', UNAIDS Case Study, July.

UNAIDS (2000b) 'Collaboration with Traditional Healers in HIV/AIDS Prevention and Care in Sub-Saharan Africa: A Literature Review', UNAIDS Best Practise Collection, Key Documents.

UNAIDS (2004) 'Facing the Future Together', Report of the United Nations Secretary-General's Task Force on Women, Girls and HIV/AIDS in Southern Africa.

UNAIDS (2005) 'Resource Needs for an Expanded Response to AIDS in Low and Middle Income Countries', Discussion Paper, London, 9 March <http://data.unaids.org/UNA-docs/three-ones_financing_en.pdf>.

UNAIDS (2007) 'Taking Action against HIV: A Handbook for Parliamentarians', Handbook for Parliamentarians, Number 15.

UNAIDS (2008a) 'Sub-Saharan Africa AIDS Epidemic Update – Regional Summary', United Nations Programme on HIV/AIDS (UNAIDS) Report, March.

UNAIDS (2008b) 'Report on the Global AIDS Epidemic', UNAIDS Report <http://data.unaids.org/pub/GlobalReport/2008/JC1511_GR08_ExecutiveSummary_en.pdf>.

UNAIDS (2008c) 'Male Circumcision and HIV Prevention in Eastern and Southern Africa', Communications Guidance.

UNAIDS (2009a) '2009: AIDS Epidemic Update', UNAIDS Report <http://data.unaids.org/pub/Report/2009/JC1700_Epi_Update_2009_en.pdf>.

UNAIDS (2009b) 'What Countries Need: Investments Needed for 2010 Targets', Joint United Nations Programme on HIV/AIDS Paper <http://data.unaids.org/pub/Report/2009/jc1681_what_countries_need_en.pdf>.

UNCTAD (2009) 'Food Security in Africa: Learning Lessons from the Food Crisis', Trade and Development Board Report TD/B/EX(47)/3, 21 April <http://www.unctad.org/en/docs/tdbex47d3_en.pdf>.

UNDP (2006) *Human Development Report 2006: Beyond Scarcity – Power, Poverty and the Global Water Crisis* (Basingstoke: Palgrave Macmillan).

UNDP (2008) 'Human Development Indices: A Statistical Update 2008', Human Development Report, December, <http://hdr.undp.org/en/media/HDI_2008_EN_Tables.pdf>.

USAID (2000) 'USAID Combating AIDS: A Record of Accomplishment', US Agency for International Development, Fact Sheet, 9 July <http://www.usaid.gov/press/releases/2000/aids_accomp.html>.

US Government (1996) 'Addressing the Threat of Emerging Infectious Diseases', The White House Office of Science and Technology Policy, Fact Sheet, 12 June.

US Government (1999) 'A National Security Strategy for a New Century', The White House, December.

US Government (2002) 'The National Security Strategy of the United States of America', White House, September.

US Government (2003a) 'United States Leadership against HIV/AIDS, Tuberculosis and Malaria Act', One Hundred Eighth Congress of the United States of America: House of Representatives.

US Government (2003b) 'President Delivers "State of the Union"', White House Office of the Press Secretary, 28 January.

US Government (2003c) 'George Bush Delivers Commencement Address at Coast Guard', White House Office of the Press Secretary, 21 May.

US Government (2003d) 'Remarks by the President on the Signing of H.R. 1298, the US Leadership Against HIV/AIDS, Tuberculosis and Malaria Act of 2003', White House Office of the Press Secretary, 27 May.

US Government (2003e) 'World AIDS Day, 2003', White House Office of the Press Secretary, 1 December.

US Government (2004) 'President Bush Discusses HIV/AIDS Initiatives in Philadelphia', White House Office of the Press Secretary, 23 June.

US Government (2006) 'The National Security Strategy of the United States of America', White House, March.

US Government (2007) 'President Bush Discusses World AIDS Day', White House Office of the Press Secretary, 30 November.

US Government (2008a) 'President and Mrs Bush Discuss Africa Policy', White House Office of the Press Secretary, 14 February.

US Government (2008b) 'President Bush Discusses Trip to Africa at Leon H. Sullivan Foundation', White House Office of the Press Secretary, 26 February.

US Government (2008c) 'President Bush Meets with President Museveni of Uganda', White House Press Release, 23 September.

van den Bout-van den Beukel, C. J. P., Koopmans, P. P., van der Ven, A. J. A. M., De Smet, P. A. G. M. and Burger, D. M. (2006) 'Possible Drug-Metabolism Interactions of Medicinal Herbs with Antiretroviral Agents', *Drug Metabolism Reviews*, 38(3): 477–514.

Van Heuverswyn, F. and Peters, M. (2007) 'The Origins of HIV and Implications for the Global Epidemic', *Current Infectious Disease Reports*, 9(4): 338–46.

van Niekerk, J. (2003) 'Failing Our Future: Responding to the Sexual Abuse of Children', *SA Crime Quarterly*, 3, March: 11–16.

Vaughan, M. (1991) *Curing Their Ills: Colonial Power and African Illness* (Cambridge: Polity Press).

Vetten, L. and Bhana, K. (2001) 'Violence, Vengeance and Gender: A Preliminary Investigation into the Links between Violence against Women and HIV/AIDS in South Africa', Centre for the Study of Violence and Reconciliation.

Vetten, L. and Haffejee, S. (2005) 'Gang Rape: A Study in Inner-City Johannesburg', *South African Crime Quarterly*, 12: 31–6.

Vetten, L., Jewkes, R., Sigsworth, R., Christofides, N., Loots, L. and Dunseith, O. (2008) 'Tracking Justice: The Attrition of Rape Cases through the Criminal Justice System in Gauteng', Johannesburg: Tshwaranang Legal Advocacy Centre, the South African Medical Research Council and the Centre for the Study of Violence and Reconciliation.

Vincent, L. (2008) 'Cutting Tradition: The Political Regulation of Traditional Circumcision Rites in South Africa's Liberal Democratic Order', *Journal of Southern African Studies*, 34(1): 77–91.

Vincent, L. (2009) 'Moral Panic and the Politics of Populism', *Representation*, 45(2): 213–21.

Walker, R. (2009) 'A New and Improved PEPFAR under Obama?', *PlusNews*, 21 January <http://www.irinnews.org/Report.aspx?ReportId=82494#>.

Wang, J. (2008) 'AIDS Denialism and "The Humanisation of the African"', *Race and Class*, 49(3): 1–18.

Wawer, M. J., Gray, R., Serwadda, D., Namukwaya, Z., Makumbi, F., Sewankambo, N., Li, X., Lutalo, T., Nalugoda, F. and Quinn, T. (2005) 'Declines in HIV Prevalence in Uganda: Not as Simple as ABC', 12th Conference on Retroviruses and Opportunistic Infections, Boston Massachusetts, 22–25 February, Abstract <http://www.retroconference.org/2005/CD/Abstracts/25775.htm>.

Waxman, H. A. (2006) 'Pharmaceutical Industry Profits Increase by over $8 Billion after Medicare Drug Plan goes into Effect', Committee on Government Reform, US House of Representatives, September.

Waxman, H. A. (2008) 'HIV/AIDS Today', *Committee on Oversight and Government Reform*, 1(5), February 15.

Weiss, R. A. (2001a) 'Natural and Iatrogenic Factors in Human Immunodeficiency Virus Transmission', *The Royal Society, Philosophical Transactions B*, 356(1410): 947–53.

Weiss, R. A. (2001b) 'The Leeuwenhoek Lecture 2001: Animal Origins of Human Infectious Disease', *The Royal Society, Philosophical Transactions B*, 356(1410): 957–77.

Weiss, R. A. (2003) 'Concluding Remarks: Emerging Persistent Infections – Family Heirlooms and New Acquisitions', Paper presented at the Origin of HIV and Emerging Persistent Viruses, Rome.

White, M. (2006) 'Drug Patents are Good for Our Health', PhRMA Press Release, 4 January.

Whiteside, A. and Sunter, C. (2000) *AIDS: The Challenge for South Africa* (Cape Town: Human & Rousseau).

WHO (1976) 'Traditional Medicine and Its Role in the Development of Health Services in Africa', Paper prepared for World Health Organization Regional Committee for Africa, 26th Session, Kampala, September.

WHO (1986) 'Acquired Immunodeficiency Syndrome (AIDS): WHO/CDC Case Definition for AIDS', *Weekly Epidemiological Record*, 61(10): 69–76.

WHO (1990) 'Report of the Consultation on AIDS and Traditional Medicine: Prospects for Involving Traditional Health Practitioners', Francistown, Botswana, WHO/TRM/GPA/90.1, 23–27 July.

WHO (1995) 'An Overview of Selected Curable Sexually Transmitted Diseases', WHO Initiative on HIV/AIDS and Sexually Transmitted Infections (HSI), Global Programme on AIDS.

WHO (2000) 'The World Health Report 2000 – Health Systems: Improving Performance', WHO Annual Report.

WHO (2001) 'Water-Related Diseases', Water Sanitation and Health (WSH) Fact Sheet <http://www.who.int/water_sanitation_health/diseases/malnutrition/en/>.

WHO (2002) 'WHO Traditional Medicine Strategy 2002–2005', WHO/EDM/TRM/2002.1.

WHO (2003) 'Unsafe Injection Practices and HIV Infection', Meeting Summary, Geneva, 14 March <http://www.who.int/hiv/strategic/mt14303/en/index.html>.

WHO (2003) 'Gender and HIV/AIDS', Gender and Health Paper, November <http://www.who.int/gender/documents/en/HIV_AIDS.pdf>.

WHO (2005) 'Access to Medicines: Intellectual Property Protection: Impact on Public Health', *WHO Drug Information*, 19(3): 236–41.

WHO (2006a) 'Working Together for Health: The World Health Report 2006', WHO Annual Report.

WHO (2006b) 'Facts about Health in the African Region of WHO', World Health Organisation Fact Sheet No. 314 <http://www.who.int/mediacentre/fact-sheets/fs314/en/index.html>.

WHO (2006c) 'Traditional Medicine Promotion', *Asia-Pacific Tech Monitor*, November–December.

WHO (2007a) 'Towards Universal Access: Scaling Up Priority HIV/AIDS Interventions in the Health Sector', Progress Report, April.

WHO (2007b) 'Prioritizing Second-Line Antiretroviral Drugs for Adults and Adolescents: A Public Health Approach', Report of a WHO Working Group Meeting, 21–22 May.

WHO (2008a) 'Towards Universal Access: Scaling Up Priority HIV/AIDS Interventions in the Health Sector', Progress Report, April.

WHO (2008b) 'Traditional Medicine', Fact Sheet Number 134, December.

WHO (2008c) 'Primary Health Care (Now More Than Ever)', The World Health Report 2008.

WHO (2009a) 'Yaws: A Forgotten Disease', Fact Sheet <http://www.who.int/neglected_diseases/diseases/yaws/en/print.html>

WHO (2009b) 'Transaction Prices for Antiretroviral Medicines and HIV Diagnostics from 2008 to April 2009', A Summary Report from the Global Price Reporting Mechanism, June.

WHO (2009c) 'Health Workforce, Infrastructure, Essential Medicines: World Health Statistics 2009', World Health Organisation Statistical Report.

WHO (2009d) 'AIDS and HIV Case Definitions: Overview of Internationally Used HIV/AIDS Case Definitions', World Health Organisation Strategic Information <http://www.who.int/hiv/strategic/surveillance/definitions/en/>.

WHO (2009e) 'World Health Statistics 2009', WHO Statistical Information System Report <http://www.who.int/whosis/whostat/EN_WHS09_Table7.pdf>.

WHO (2009f) 'Traditional Medicine in the WHO African Region' <http://www.info.gov.za/events/2009/trad_medicine.pdf>.

WHO (2009g) 'Towards Universal Access: Scaling Up Priority HIV/AIDS Interventions in the Health Sector', Progress Report.

WHO (2010a) 'More Information about PEP for HIV Prevention', WHO Fact Sheet <http://www.who.int/hiv/topics/prophylaxis/info/en/>.

WHO (2010b) 'Prequalification', World Health Organisation, Health Topics <http://www.who.int/topics/prequalification/en/>.

Willcox, B. W. (2008) 'A Scientific Review of Abstinence and Abstinence Programs', Technical Assistance Module for Abstinence Education Grantees: Pal-Tech, Inc.

Willcox, R. R. (1946) 'Venereal Disease in West Africa', *Nature*, 157: 416–19.

Witwer, K (2007) 'Science Outsold? Correcting the Falsehoods of Science Sold Out: Does HIV Really Cause AIDS by Dr Rebecca V Culshaw', AIDSTruth Paper, April.

Worcester, R. (2006) 'Public Attitudes towards Science: What do We Know', in Turney, J. (ed.) *Engaging Science: Thoughts, Deeds, Analysis and Action* (London: The Wellcome Trust).

World Bank (2004) 'Indigenous Knowledge: Local Pathways to Global Development', Report Marking Five Years of the World Bank Indigenous Knowledge for Development Programme, Knowledge and Learning Group, Africa Region.

World Bank (2007) 'People', in *World Development Indicators 2007* (Washington DC: World Bank).

WRD (2008) *World Religion Database – International Religious Demographic Statistics and Sources* (Boston: Brill).

Wreford, J. (2005) 'Negotiating Relationships between Biomedicine and Sangoma: Fundamental Misunderstandings, Avoidable Mistakes', CSSR Working Paper, Number 138, December.

Wreford, J. (2008a) 'Myths, Masks and Stark Realities: Traditional African Healers, HIV/AIDS Narratives and Patterns of HIV/AIDS Avoidance', CSSR Working Paper, Number 209, January.

Wreford, J. (2008b) 'Shaming and Blaming: Medical Myths, Traditional Health Practitioners and HIV/AIDS in South Africa', CSSR Working Paper Number 211, January.

WTO (1994) 'Annex 1C: Trade-Related Aspects of Intellectual Property Rights (TRIPS)', Agreement Establishing the World Trade Organization <http://www.wto.org/english/docs_e/legal_e/27-trips.pdf>.

WTO (2001) 'Declaration on the TRIPS Agreement and Public Health', Ministerial Conference, Fourth Session, Doha, 9–14 November.

WTO (2003) 'Decision Removes Final Patent Obstacle to Cheap Drug Imports', Press Release, Press/350/Rev.1, 30 August.

WTO (2008) *Understanding the WTO*, Fourth Edition (Geneva: WTO Publications).

WWF (2002) 'Water in Africa', Fact Sheet, July <http://assets.panda.org/downloads/waterinafricaeng.pdf>.

Young, A. (2004) 'The Gift of Dying: The Tragedy of AIDS and the Welfare of Future African Generations', *Quarterly Journal of Economics*, 120(2): 423–66.

Yusim, K., Peeters, M., Pybus, O. G., Bhattacharya, T., Delaporte, E., Mulanga, C., Muldoon, M., Theiler, J. and Korber, B. (2001) 'Using Human Immunodeficiency Virus Type 1 Sequences to Infer Historical Features of the Acquired Immune Deficiency Syndrome Epidemic and Human Immunodeficiency Virus Evolution', *The Royal Society, Philosophical Transactions B*, 356(1410): 855–66.

Zinn, H. (1990) *The Politics of History*, Second Edition (Illinois: University of Illinois Press).

Zwi, A. and Bachmayer, D. (1990) 'HIV and AIDS in South Africa: What is an Appropriate Public Health Response?', *Health Policy and Planning*, 5(4): 316–26.

Zwi, A. B. and Cabral, A. J. R. (1991) 'Identifying "High Risk Situations" for Preventing AIDS', *British Medical Journal*, 303(6816): 1527–9.

Zwillich, T. (2009) 'Obama Administration may Flat-line Funding for PEPFAR', *The Lancet*, 373(9672): 1325.

Index